Life or Death—
Who Controls?

Nancy C. Ostheimer brings to her role of co-editor of *Life or Death—Who Controls?* the timely attributes of the involved citizen who is also a keen observer of the sociopolitical scene. A writer by profession, she shares the concern of her husband and collaborator for the controversial human issues of our day.

John M. Ostheimer is currently associate professor of political science at Northern Arizona University, where he has taught since 1967. Previously he was for two years on the faculty of the University of Dar Es Salaam, in Tanzania. Dr. Ostheimer, who received his Ph.D. from Yale University, has published a number of articles on environmental problems and sociopolitical developments in Africa, as well as two books, *Nigerian Politics* and *Politics of the Western Indian Ocean Islands*.

Life or Death—
Who Controls?

EDITED BY

Nancy C. Ostheimer
John M. Ostheimer

Springer Publishing Company/New York

Springer Publishing Company, Inc.
200 Park Avenue South
New York, N.Y. 10003

Library of Congress Cataloging in Publication Data

Main entry under title:

Life or death—who controls?

    Bibliography: p.
    Includes index.
    1. Bioethics. 2. Medical ethics
I. Ostheimer, Nancy C. II. Ostheimer, John M.
[DNLM: 1. Abortion, Induced. 2. Euthanasia.
3. Eugenics. 4. Ethics, Medical. W50 L722]
QH332.L53   174'.2   75-31522
ISBN 0-8261-2020-2
ISBN 0-8261-2021-0

Printed in U.S.A.

Contents

Part III Compulsory Sterilization: Population Control or Genocide? 161

Part IV How to Die: Euthanasia 213

Preface

Virtually all of the predominant religious and ethical values in Western societies stress the dignity and preservation of human life. Nothing is considered more sacred. Technologically, the means of sustaining life, even of creating it, offer an ever-widening set of options. At the same time there are many arguments against using modern science to preserve life: the gnawing economic and demographic imperatives of postindustrial societies; the realization that trying to defeat fatal illnesses is prohibitively painful as well as useless beyond a certain point; the possibility that humanity is undergoing physiological decline as the impact of natural selection is circumvented; ethnic fears that medical technology will be used for "genocidal" purposes. Thus many people are arguing that societies should not employ "miraculous" technology just because it exists.

In any case, thanks to technology, advanced societies are increasingly able to interfere with standard patterns of birth and death. This common thread holds together such apparently diverse issues as abortion, eugenic manipulation, euthanasia, and compulsory sterilization—issues in which society is called to make "life or death" decisions. As the scientific capacity for such social intervention continues to grow, the inherently emotional nature of the issues guarantees that they will be of extraordinary importance in the political arena. Western societies, with their traditions of humanism, fundamental individual rights, and comparatively limited powers of government, offer unique battlegrounds for such issues. For balanced against this tradition of individual rights are the scientific and monetary arguments for biomedical policies that appear to benefit society by saving welfare funds, by lowering crime rates, or by improving the prospects of population control.

This anthology is designed to provide an introductory treatment of life-and-death issues. We have no cause to espouse, and have tried to select writings that display the range of arguments on each issue. As will become obvious, the issues are related by a single theme: the need to make certain social, and ultimately political, choices. By bringing together such diverse opinions, we hope to give our readers a basis for making these choices in an informed, intelligent manner.

Contributors

Frank J. Ayd, Jr. is a medical doctor in Baltimore, Maryland. He edits and publishes *The Medical-Moral Newsletter.*

Carl Jay Bajema is professor of biology at Grand Valley State College, Allendale, Michigan, and has recently been a visiting professor of anthropology at Harvard University.

Mildred B. Beck was formerly Acting Chief, Office of Information, National Center for Family Planning Services, Health Services and Mental Health Administration, U.S. Department of Health, Education, and Welfare, Rockville, Maryland.

David Dempsey is a freelance writer living in Rye, New York.

Paul R. Ehrlich is professor of biological sciences at Stanford University, Stanford, California. Co-author Anne is a writer.

Darrel S. English is associate professor of genetics at Northern Arizona University, Flagstaff.

Joseph Fletcher is Visiting Professor of Medical Ethics at the University of Virginia, Charlottesville.

Charles Frankel is Old Dominion Professor of Philosophy and Public Affairs at Columbia University, New York City.

Jan Charles Gray is a member of the California and District of Columbia Bars.

Frederic Grunberg is associate professor of psychiatry at Albany Medical College of Union University.

Garrett Hardin is professor of biology and human ecology at the University of California at Santa Barbara.

Kurt Hirschhorn is professor of pediatrics (genetics) and Chief,

Division of Medical Genetics, at Mount Sinai School of Medicine in New York City.

Donald Huisingh is associate professor of plant pathology at North Carolina State University at Raleigh.

Elisabeth Kübler-Ross is a writer and medical doctor who has done extensive research on elderly and terminal patients.

Richard Landau is a former Ohio newspaperman and is now at Tufts University.

Marya Mannes is a novelist, essayist, and critic. She has written for numerous national publications and appears frequently on television.

Richard A. McCormick, S.J. is Rose F. Kennedy Professor of Christian Ethics at the Joseph and Rose Kennedy Institute for the Study of Human Reproduction and Bioethics, Georgetown University, Washington, D.C.

Victor K. McElheny is a reporter for *The New York Times.*

John A. Miles, Jr. is in the department of theology, Loyola University, Chicago.

John T. Noonan, Jr. is professor of law at the University of California Law School at Berkeley.

Leonard G. Ritt is assistant professor of political science at Northern Arizona University, Flagstaff.

Hyman Rodman is Excellence Fund Professor, Child Development and Family Relations, at the University of North Carolina at Greensboro.

Betty Sarvis was a research assistant at the Merrill-Palmer Institute during the time *The Abortion Controversy* was written.

Jack Slater, a former staff writer for *Ebony* magazine, is now an editor at *The New York Times Magazine*, where he writes on the arts and on general topics.

Nick Thimmesch is a syndicated columnist for *Newsday,* and is based in Washington, D.C.

Life or Death—
Who Controls?

Part I

Eugenics: Social Choice or Nature's Way?

"Test tube babies alive in England" read the headlines, but to many biomedical success is a transgression of the human role: the ability to create life only strengthens man's arrogance at the very time the human race must learn the humility of living within the world's limits.

Should mankind interfere in the "natural" processes of life? To what degree, and under what conditions? Part 1 includes a variety of outlooks on such questions, and, as the selections clearly reveal, there seems to be little consensus in the public mind.

Carl Jay Bajema fears that the next generation will have a larger proportion of harmful genes and discusses various methods of population control for both quality and quantity.

Charles Frankel is quite sceptical of genetic manipulation. He argues that we do not know enough about the future to judge which genetic traits will be useful.

Some background to the issues is provided by Darrel S. English, who cautions that all implications (moral, ethical, and so on) must be considered when discussing genetic manipulation for society's purposes. This sense of caution is underlined by a *New York Times* article announcing the decision of some scientists to suspend such research until the hazards are fully known. In contrast to this is the selection from Joseph Fletcher's book *The Ethics of Genetic Control,* encouraging experiments in genetic intervention in order to prevent disease and disfigurement. Kurt Hirschhorn warns that we cannot significantly improve the human race through genetic intervention and still allow for evolutionary improvement. Hirschhorn believes that population control can be made to serve as a quality control measure.

One key issue remains for discussion: Is there a real need to improve the gene pool? Donald Huisingh argues that we do not now use the genetic potential that we *have*. Huisingh thinks that we should concentrate on improving educational opportunities so that we can develop the intellectual capabilities that already exist.

1

The Genetic Implications
of Population Control

Carl Jay Bajema

Introduction

Each generation of mankind is faced with the awesome responsibility of having to make decisions concerning the quantity and quality (both genetic and cultural) of future generations. Because of its concern for its increasing population in relation to natural resources and quality of life, America appears to be on the verge of discarding its policy favoring continued population growth and adopting a policy aimed at achieving a zero rate of population growth by voluntary means. The policy that a society adopts with respect to population size will have genetic as well as environmental consequences.

Human populations adapt to their environments genetically as well as culturally (Bajema, 1971). These environments have been and are changing very rapidly, with most of the changes being brought about by man himself. Mankind has, by creating a highly technological society, produced a society in which a significant proportion of its citizens cannot contribute to its growth or maintenance because of the limitations (both genetic and environmental) of their intellect. The modern technological societies of democratic nations offer their citizens a wide variety of opportunities for self-fulfillment but find that many of their citizens are incapable of taking advantage of the opportunities open to them.

American society, if it takes its responsibility to future generations seriously, will have to do more than control the size of

From *Bioscience* 21 (January 15, 1971), pp. 71-75. Reprinted by permission of the American Institute of Biological Sciences and the author.

This is an expanded version of a working paper prepared for the First National Congress on Optimum Population and Environment, Chicago, June 7-11, 1970.

its population in relation to the environment. American society will have to take steps to insure that individuals yet unborn will have the best genetic and environmental heritage possible to enable them to meet the challenges of the environment and to be able to take advantage of the opportunities for self-fulfillment made available by society.

The question of genetic quality cannot be ignored for very long by American society because it, like all other human societies, has to cope with two perpetual problems as it attempts to adapt to its environment. First, American society has to cope with a continual input of harmful genes into its population via mutation (it has been estimated that approximately one out of every five newly fertilized human eggs is carrying a newly mutated gene that was not present in either of the two parents). The genetic status quo can be maintained in a human population only if the number of new mutant genes added to the population is counterbalanced by an equal number of the mutant genes not being passed on due to the nonreproduction or decreased reproduction of individuals carrying these mutant genes. Otherwise, the proportion of harmful genes in the population will increase. Second, American society has to adapt to a rapidly changing environment. For instance, the technologically-based, sociocultural, computer age environment being created by American society has placed a premium on the possession of high intelligence and creativity. Our society requires individuals with high intelligence and creativity to help it make the appropriate social and technological adjustments in order to culturally adapt to its rapidly changing environment. On the other hand, individuals require high intelligence and creativity in order that they, as individuals, can cope with the challenges of the environment and take advantage of the opportunities for self-fulfillment present in our society.

The proportion of the American population that already is genetically handicapped—that suffers a restriction of liberty or competence because of the genes they are carrying—is not small. Therefore the genetic component of the human population-environment equation must be taken into account as we attempt to establish an environment that has a high degree of ecological stability and that maximizes the number of opportunities for self-fulfillment available to each individual human being.

*Genetic Consequences of American Life Styles
in Sex and Reproduction*

American life styles with respect to sex and reproduction are
currently in a tremendous state of flux and are changing rapidly.
This makes it very difficult to accurately predict the genetic
consequences of these life styles. Yet, because these life styles
determine the genetic make-up of future generations of Americans, it is necessary that we evaluate the genetic consequences of
past and present trends and speculate concerning the probable
genetic consequences of projecting these trends into the future.
Only then will we be able to determine the severity of the problem
and to determine what steps, if any, need to be taken to maintain
and improve the genetic heritage of future generations.

American society has developed modern medical techniques
which enable many individuals with severe genetic defects to
survive to adulthood. Many of these individuals can and do
reproduce, thereby passing their harmful genes on to the next
generation and increasing the frequency of these genes in the
population. At present, there is no indication that heredity
counseling decreases the probability that these individuals will
have children. The life styles of these individuals with respect to
reproduction is creating a larger genetic burden for future
generations of Americans to bear.

The effect of American life styles in sex and reproduction on
such behavioral patterns as intelligence and personality is much
less clear. For instance, during most of man's evolution natural
selection has favored the genes for intelligence. The genes for
higher mental ability conferred an advantage to their carriers in
the competition for survival and reproduction both within and
between populations. Thus the more intelligent members of the
human species passed more genes on to the next generation than
did the less intelligent members, with the result that the genes for
higher intelligence increased in frequency. As Western societies
shifted from high birth and death rates toward low birth and death
rates, however, a breakdown in the relation of natural selection to
achievement or "success" took place.

The practice of family planning spread more rapidly among the
better educated strata of society resulting in negative fertility
differentials. At the period of extreme differences, which in the
United States came during the Great Depression, the couples who

were poorly educated were having about twice as many children as the more educated couples. The continued observation of a negative relationship between fertility and such characteristics as education, occupation, and income during the first part of this century led many scientists to believe that this pattern of births was a concomitant of the industrial welfare state society and must make for the genetic deterioration of the human race. This situation was, in part, temporary. The fertility differentials have declined dramatically since World War II so that by the 1960s some women college graduates were having 90% as many children as the U.S. average (Kirk, 1969). A number of recent studies of American life styles in reproduction, when taken collectively, seem to indicate that, as the proportion of the urban population raised in a farm environment decreases, as the educational attainment of the population increases, and as women gain complete control over childbearing (via contraception and induced abortion), the relationship between fertility and such characteristics as income, occupation, and educational attainment will become less negative and may even become positive (Goldberg, 1959, 1960, 1965; Freedman and Slesinger, 1961; Duncan, 1965).

The only two American studies which have related the intellectual ability (as measured by IQ) of an individual to his subsequent completed fertility have found the relationship to be essentially zero or slightly positive (Bajema, 1963; Waller, 1969). Further analyses of the data of these two studies indicate that it is difficult to infer the relationship between intelligence (as measured by IQ) and fertility from group differences in fertility with respect to income, occupation, and educational attainment because there is so much variation within these groups with respect to intelligence (Bajema, 1966, 1968; Waller, 1969).

The overall net effect of current American life styles in reproduction appears to be slightly dysgenic—to be favoring an increase in harmful genes which will genetically handicap a larger proportion of the next generation of Americans. American life styles in reproduction are, in part, a function of the population policy of the United States. What will be the long-range genetic implications of controlling or not controlling population size in an industrialized welfare state democracy such as America?

Genetic Implications of Policies Favoring Control of Population Growth

Most contemporary human societies are organized in such a way that they encourage population growth. How is the genetic make-up of future generations affected by the size of the population? What will be the ultimate genetic consequences given a society that is growing in numbers in relation to its environment? One possible consequence is military aggression coupled with genocide to attain additional living space. This would result in genetic change insofar as the population eradicated or displaced differs genetically from the population that is aggressively expanding the size of its environment. The displacement of the American Indians by West Europeans is an example of this approach to the problem of population size in relation to the environment (Hulse, 1961). Throughout man's evolution such competition between different populations of human beings has led to an increase in the cultural and genetic supports for aggressive behavior in the human species. Violence as a form of aggressive behavior to solve disagreements among populations appears to have become mal-adaptive in the nuclear age. It will probably take a nuclear war to prove this contention.

If one assumes that military aggression plus genocide to attain additional living space is not an option open to a society with a population policy encouraging growth in numbers then a different type of genetic change will probably take place. Most scientists who have attempted to ascertain the probable effect that overcrowding in a welfare state will have on man's genetic make-up have concluded that natural selection would favor those behavior patterns that most people consider least desirable. For instance, Rene Dubos (1965), in discussing the effect of man's future environment on the direction and intensity of natural selection in relation to human personality patterns, states that:

> Most disturbing perhaps are the behavioral consequences likely to ensue from overpopulation. The everincreasing complexity of the social structure will make some form of regimentation unavoidable; freedom and privacy may come to constitute antisocial luxuries and their attainment to involve real hardships. In consequence, there may emerge by selection a stock of human beings suited to accept as a matter

of course a regimented and sheltered way of life in a teeming and polluted world, from which all wilderness and fantasy of nature will have disappeared. The domesticated farm animal and the laboratory rodent in a controlled environment will then become true models for the study of man.

The genetic and cultural undesirability of either of these two alternative outcomes for mankind makes it imperative that societies move quickly to adopt policies aimed at achieving and maintaining an optimum population size that maximizes the dignity and individual worth of a human being rather than maximizing the number of human beings in relation to the environment.

Genetic Implications of Policies Favoring Control of Population Size by Voluntary Means

There is strong evidence that contemporary societies can achieve control of their population size by voluntary means, at least in the short run.

What will be the distribution of births in societies that have achieved a zero population growth rate? In a society where population size is constant—where each generation produces only enough offspring to replace itself—there will still be variation among couples with respect to the number of children they will have. Some individuals will be childless or have only one child for a variety of reasons—biological (genetically or environmentally caused sterility), psychological (inability to attract a mate, desire to remain childless), etc. Some individuals will have to have at least three children to compensate for those individuals who have less than two children. The resulting differential fertility—variation in the number of children couples have—provides an opportunity for natural selection to operate and would bring about genetic change if the differences in fertility among individuals are correlated with differences (physical, physiological, or behavioral) among individuals.

The United States is developing into a social welfare state democracy. This should result in an environment that will evoke the optimal response from the variety of genotypes (specific combinations of genes that individuals carry) present in the population. It is questionable, however, as to whether a social welfare state democracy creates the type of environment that will automatically bring about a eugenic distribution of births resulting in the maintenance or enhancement of man's genetic heritage. It is also questionable as to whether a social welfare state democracy (or any society for that matter) will be able to achieve and maintain a zero population growth rate—a constant population size—by voluntary means.

Both Charles Darwin (1958) and Garrett Hardin (1968) have argued that universal compulsion will be necessary to achieve and maintain zero population growth. They argue that appeals to individual conscience as the means by which couples are to restrain themselves from having more than two children will not work because those individuals or groups who refused to restrain themselves would increase their numbers in relation to the rest, with the result that these individuals or groups with their cultural and/or biological supports for high fertility would constitute a larger and larger proportion of the population of future generations and *Homo contracipiens* would be replaced by *Homo progenetivis*.

Hardin (1968) raises this problem in his classic paper, "The Tragedy of the Commons," when he states:

> If each human family were dependent only on its own resources; if the children of improvident parents starved to death; if, thus, overbreeding brought its own "punishment" to the germ line—then there would be no public interest in controlling the breeding of families. But our society is deeply committed to the welfare state, and hence confronted with another aspect of the tragedy of the commons.
>
> In a welfare state, how shall we deal with the family, the religion, the race, or the class (or indeed any distinguishable and cohesive group) that adopts overbreeding as a policy to secure its own aggrandizement? To couple the concept of freedom to breed with the belief that everyone born has an equal right to the commons is to lock the world into a tragic course of action.

The only way out of this dilemma according to Hardin is for society to create reproductive responsibility via social arrangements that produce coercion of some sort. The kind of coercion Hardin talks about is mutual coercion, mutually agreed upon by the majority of the people affected. Compulsory taxes are an example of mutual coercion. Democratic societies frequently have to resort to mutual coercion to escape destruction of the society by the irresponsible. Mutual coercion appears to be the only solution to the problem of pollution. If Hardin is right, it may also be the only solution for any society that is attempting to control the size and/or the genetic make-up of its population.

Hardin's thesis has been questioned on the basis that children are no longer the economic assets they once were in agrarian societies. Rufous Miles has argued that, given today's postindustrial economy, children are expensive pleasures; they are economic liabilities rather than assets. Miles (1970) points out that:

> There is no conflict, therefore, between the economic self-interest of married couples to have small families and the collective need of society to preserve "the commons." It is in both their interests to limit procreation to not more than a replacement level. Unfortunately, couples do not seek their self-interest in economic terms alone, but in terms of total satisfactions. They are "buying" children and paying dearly for them. The problem, therefore, is compounded of how to persuade couples to act more in their own economic self-interest and that of their children; how to assist them in obtaining more psychological satisfactions from sources other than large families; and how to replace the outworn and now inimical tradition of the large family with a new "instant tradition" of smaller families.

As pointed out earlier in this paper, there is some evidence to support the contention that as American society becomes more urbanized, achieves higher levels of educational attainment, and allows its citizens to exercise complete control over their fertility, reproductive patterns will develop which will lead to a zero or negative population growth rate and a eugenic distribution of births. If this prediction is correct, then there will be no need for the adoption of mutual coercion—compulsory methods of population control—by American society in order to control the size and/or genetic quality of its population. If, on the other hand, these reproductive patterns do not develop or are transitory, it may very well be that reproduction will have to become a privilege rather than a right in social welfare state democracies in order to insure that these societies and their citizens do not have to suffer the environmental and genetic consequences of irresponsible reproduction.

What might the genetic consequences be if a society had to

resort to mutual coercion—had to employ compulsory methods of population control—to control its numbers?

Genetic Implications of Compulsory Population Control

There are a number of methods by which compulsory population control can be achieved (Berelson, 1969). Mutual coercion could be institutionalized by a democratic society to ensure that couples who would otherwise be reproductively irresponsible are restricted to having only two children. Compulsory abortion and/or sterilization could be employed to guarantee that no woman bears more children than she has a right to under the rules set up by society.

A democratic society forced to employ mutual coercion to achieve zero population growth will probably assign everyone the right to have exactly two children. Because of the fact that some individuals will have only one child or will not reproduce at all, it will be necessary to assign these births needed to achieve replacement level to other individuals in that population. The assignment of these births could be made at random via a national lottery system. The result would probably be genetic deterioration. While those individuals who have less than two children would constitute a sample of the population with above average frequencies of various genetic defects, the selective removal of their genes would probably not be sufficient to counterbalance the continual input of mutations. Thus the result would probably be genetic deterioration even if the environment remained constant. If the environment were changing (this is about the one thing we can always count on—a constantly changing environment), the population would become even more genetically ill-adapted because those individuals in the society that are best adapted to changing environments and to the new environments would not be passing more genes on to the next generation on a per person basis than those individuals less well adapted.

What kinds of eugenics programs could be designed for a democratic society where mutual coercion is institutionalized to ensure that couples who would otherwise be irresponsible are restricted to having two children?

One compulsory population control program designed to operate in a democratic society that has eugenic implications is the granting of marketable licenses to have children to women in whatever number necessary to ensure replacement of the population (say 2.2 children per couple). The unit certificate might be the deci-child or 1/10 a child and the accumulation of ten of these units, by purchase or inheritance or gift, would permit a woman in maturity to have one child. If equality of opportunity were the norm in such a society, those individuals with genetic make-ups that enable them to succeed (high intelligence, personality, etc.) would be successful in reaching the upper echelons of society and would be in the position of being able to purchase certificates from the individuals who were less successful because of their genetic limitations. The marketable baby license approach to compulsory population control, first discussed by Kenneth Boulding (1964) in his book *The Meaning of the Twentieth Century,* relies on the environment, especially the sociocultural environment, to do the selecting automatically, based on economics. The marketable baby license approach would probably bring about a better genetic adaptation between a population and its environment. Remember, the direction and rate of genetic change is to a great extent a function of the social structure of the human population. The marketable baby license approach ensures that those people selected in society are those who are most successful economically. To ensure genetic improvement society would have to make sure that achievement and financial reward are much more highly correlated than they are at the present.

Another compulsory population program that a democracy might adopt would be to grant each individual the right to have two children and to assign the child-bearing rights of those individuals unable or unwilling to have two children to other individuals based on their performance in one or more contests (competition involving mental ability, personality, sports, music, arts, literature, business, etc.). The number of births assigned to the winners of various contests would be equal to the deficit of births created by individuals having less than two children. Society would then determine to a great extent the direction of its future genetic (and cultural) evolution by determining the types of contests that would be employed and what proportion of the winners (the top 1% or 5%) would be rewarded with the right to have an additional child above the two children granted to all members of society.

A society might even go further and employ a simple eugenic test—the examination of the first two children in order to assure that neither one was physically or mentally below average—which a couple must pass before being eligible to have additional children (Glass, 1967). The assignment of additional births to those individuals who passed the eugenic tests then could be on the basis of a lottery, marketable baby licenses, or contests, with the number of licenses equaling the deficit of births created by individuals who, at the end of their reproductive years (or at time of death if they died before reaching the end of their reproductive years), did not have any children or who only had one child.

The programs designed to bring about a eugenic distribution of births that have been discussed so far may prove to be incapable of doing much more than counteracting the input of harmful mutations. In order to significantly reduce the proportion of the human population that is genetically handicapped, a society may have to require that each couple pass certain eugenic tests before being allowed to become the genetic parents of *any* children. If one or both of the prospective genetic parents fail the eugenic tests, the couple could still be allowed to have children via artificial insemination and/or artificial inovulation, utilizing human sperm and eggs selected on the basis of genetic quality. Such an approach would enable society to maintain the right of couples to have at least two children while improving the genetic birthright of future generations at the same time.

Successful control of the size and/or genetic quality of human populations by society may require restrictions on the right of individual human beings to reproduce. The right of individuals to have as many children as they desire must be considered in relation to the right of individuals yet unborn to be free from genetic handicaps and to be able to live in a high-quality environment. The short-term gain in individual freedom attained in a society that grants everyone the right to reproduce and to have as many children as they want can be more than offset by the long-term loss in individual freedom by individuals yet unborn who, as a consequence, are genetically handicapped and/or are forced to live in an environment that has deteriorated due to the pressure of human numbers.

Conclusion

Each generation of mankind faces anew the awesome responsibility of making decisions which will affect the quantity and genetic quality of the next generation. A society, if it takes its responsibility to future generations seriously, will take steps to ensure that individuals yet unborn will have the best genetic and cultural heritage possible to enable them to meet the challenges of the environment and to take advantage of the opportunities for self-fulfillment present in that society.

The way in which a society is organized will determine, to a great extent, the direction and intensity of natural selection especially with respect to behavioral patterns. The genetic make-up of future generations is also a function of the size of the population and how population size is regulated by society. The genetic implications of the following three basic types of population policies were explored in this paper:

1. policies favoring continued population growth;
2. policies aimed at achieving zero population growth by voluntary means; and
3. policies aimed at achieving zero population growth by compulsory measures (mutual coercion mutually agreed upon in a democratic society).

If societies adopt compulsory population control measures, it will be for the control of population size and not for the control of the genetic make-up of the population. However, it is but a short step to compulsory control of genetic quality once compulsory programs aimed at controlling population size have been adopted. The author personally hopes that mankind will be able to solve both the quantitative and qualitative problems of population by voluntary means. Yet one must be realistic and consider the alternatives. This is what the author has attempted to do in this paper by reviewing the genetic implications of various population control programs.

References

Bajema, C. 1963. "Estimation of the Direction and Intensity of Natural Selection in Relation to Intelligence by Means of the Intrinsic Rate of Natural Increase." *Eugenics Quarterly* 10: 175-87.

_____. 1966. "Relation of Fertility to Educational Attainment in a

Kalamazoo Public School Population: A Follow-up Study." *Eugenics Quarterly* 13: 306-15.

_____. "Relation of Fertility to Occupational Status, IQ, Educational Attainment and Size of Family of Origin: A Follow-up Study of a Male Kalamazoo Public School Population." *Eugenics Quarterly* 15: 198-203.

_____, ed. 1971. *Natural Selection in Human Populations: The Measurement of Ongoing Genetic Evolution in Contemporary Human Societies.* New York: John Wiley.

Berelson, B. 1968. "Beyond Family Planning." *Science* 163: 533-43.

Boulding, K. 1964. *The Meaning of the Twentieth Century: The Great Transition.* New York: Harper & Row.

Darwin, C. 1958. *The Problems of World Population.* Cambridge: Cambridge University Press, 42 pp.

Dubos, R. 1965. *Man Adapting.* New Haven: Yale University Press.

Duncan, O. 1965. "Farm Background and Differential Fertility." *Demography* 2: 240-49.

Freedman, R., and Slesinger, D. 1961. "Fertility Differentials for the Indigenous Non-farm Population of the United States." *Population Studies* 15: 161-73.

Glass, B. 1967. "What Man Can Be." Paper presented at the American Association of School Administrators Convention, Atlantic City, N.J. 23 pp.

Goldberg, D. 1959. "The Fertility of Two-generation Urbanites." *Population Studies* 12: 214-22.

_____. 1960. "Another Look at the Indianapolis Fertility Data." *Milbank Fund Quarterly* 38: 23-36.

_____. 1965. "Fertility and Fertility Differentials: Some Observations on Recent Changes in the United States." In M. Sheps and J. Ridley, eds., *Public Health and Population Change,* Pittsburgh: University of Pittsburgh Press. pp. 119-42.

Hardin, G. 1968. "The Tragedy of the Commons." *Science* 162: 1243-48.

Hulse, F. 1961. "Warfare, Demography and Genetics." *Eugenics Quarterly* 8: 185-97.

Kirk, D. 1969. "The Genetic Implications of Family Planning." *Journal of Medical Education* 44 (Suppl. 2): 80-83.

Miles, R. 1970. "Whose Baby is the Population Problem?" *Population Bulletin* 16: 3-36.

Waller, J. 1969. "The Relationship of Fertility, Generation Length, and Social Mobility to Intelligence Test Scores, Socioeconomic Status and Educational Attainment." Doctoral thesis, University of Minnesota, Minneapolis. 100 pp.

2

The Specter of Eugenics

Charles Frankel

I

One of the often noted anomalies of our society is its capacity to
develop extraordinary new technologies while failing to find ways
to perform elementary services in a minimally decent fashion.
Nowhere is this truer, or more painful, than in medical care.
Hospitals visit tawdry indignities on patients even while their bills
reach unimaginable levels; medical services are increasingly bureau-
cratized and depersonalized; competent doctors, nurses, and
paraprofessionals are in short supply and not where they are most
needed. In these circumstances a new theme has emerged to
dominate the discussion of the moral and social responsibilities of
medicine. It is not how to humanize medicine but how to
re-engineer the human race.

The occasion for this preoccupation—which has affected the
curricula of medical and law schools, led to the creation of new
institutes and to proposed legislation in Congress,[1] and produced a
stream of sociological, moral, and philosophical reflection[2] —is the
advent of "biomedicine," a package of dazzling biological discoveries and new medical techniques. Biomedicine, we are told, is the
harbinger, or portent, of the day when man will be able to say of
himself, meaning it entirely, that, at last, he is his own greatest
creation, and has got the weight of that other Creation off his
back. Existentialist philosophers have accustomed us during the
past generation to phrases like "man invents himself." But they
have meant these dark utterances metaphorically, metaphysically.
Biomedicine, it would appear, gives them a literal meaning. If what

From *Commentary* 57 (March 1974), pp. 25-33. Copyright © 1974 by the
American Jewish Committee. Reprinted by permission of the author and
publisher.

is said about it is true, mankind is on the verge of being able to make itself, in a quite physical sense, its own principal artifact.

If what is said is true. Biomedicine has been well publicized, and all sorts of people—geneticists, doctors, theologians, philosophers, social planners—have found it personally advantageous or socially desirable to talk the subject up and paint its importance in lurid colors. One who is not a geneticist or physician must speak with diffidence, but I am not myself persuaded that all the miracles that have been announced as at hand are really about to materialize. Nevertheless, even a restrained account of recent developments will suggest why people not excessively given to utopian or apocalyptic solemnities believe that biomedicine poses unprecedented issues. Indeed, whether or not biomedicine's immediate practical significance has been exaggerated, the hopes, fears, plans, and prophecies it has provoked are themselves an illuminating avenue of entry into some of the more important fads and fallacies of current moral outlooks.

II

The excitement that biomedicine arouses begins with its fundamental achievement, the breaking of the genetic code, an accomplishment as stunning for its intellectual brilliance, and as important, in all probability, for the history of science as the first discoveries in nuclear physics. The manner in which the genes send out the "messages" that control the development of the organism is now basically understood. A large part of what used to be called "the secret of life" is therefore open for investigation, and presumably for manipulation and redesign. Human cells growing in tissue culture, for example, have been made to undergo inheritable changes when infected by a virus or treated with foreign genetic matter. To take another example, the first week of human fetal life has been reproduced entirely under laboratory conditions: sooner or later, we are told, test-tube babies will materialize.

Together with these fundamental discoveries, an array of experimental and clinical techniques has been developed that change practical perspectives on birth, maturing, aging, dying, sexuality, and the relations of parents to children, and that can alter or undermine the private rights hitherto associated with the most intimate areas of human experience. Prenatal diagnostic procedures have been discovered which permit the determination of the sex of the fetus and the presence in it of hereditary abnormalities. With the advent of legal abortion "planned parent-hood" has thus acquired a new dimension: it comprises control not simply over the number of children but over their sex and physical and mental quality. At present it is possible through prenatal diagnoses to detect sixty genetically caused defects, among which the best known and most widespread is probably mongoloidism, and it is expected that in a few years the list will be almost doubled. The advent of these diagnostic procedures has led to new ideas about the opportunities and responsibilities of preventive medicine and public-health programs. In a program of mass screening of pregnant women, for example, women diag-nosed to be carrying genetically defective children would be advised—or, in some plans, required—to take corrective action, ranging from dietary changes through chemical therapy to abortion.

Methods of genetic diagnosis are now so advanced, indeed, as to permit the envisaging of systems of universal genetic examination, instituted well before pregnancy, to permit the detecting of individuals who, although themselves healthy, are the carriers of dangerous genes in a recessive state. Such people could be advised to stay away from people of the opposite sex who carried the same recessive genes; an alternative would be to recommend that they adopt children or have them by artificial insemination. Stronger measures could also be advised or required. The suggestion has been made by advocates of compulsory population control, for example, that boys and girls be inoculated against fertility at puberty.[3] A more modest variation would be to inoculate the carriers of recessive genes for certain diseases.

By such techniques the long-range purpose of reducing the proportions of troublemaking genes in the collective human gene pool could be accomplished. The pursuit of this purpose, according to many geneticists, is an increasingly urgent imperative. The advances in medicine over the past century have decreased the significance of "natural selection" in keeping the genetic heritage of mankind relatively uncontaminated. People afflicted by inherit-able diseases live to pass them on, as do people who carry mutant genes. The result, some generations away, will be a "genetic load" of abnormalities and deficiencies painful and expensive for the species to bear. Fortunately, however, the scientific progress which has caused this problem also has presented us, it is pointed out, with the potential solution. The planned production of children is the alternative, in this perspective, to the degradation of the human stock. Nor need a sufficiently motivated society restrict itself to genetic planning for wholly negative purposes like reducing the contamination of the human gene pool. The technical capabilities already exist, enthusiasts for genetic planning point out, to set about systematically to improve the human breed. Artificial insemination using stored sperm is a well established procedure. Thus, all that is needed is a proper system of social planning, and women a hundred years from now will be able to have children by Nureyev or Henry Kissinger.

Other developments loom. In the near future, it is prophesied, it will be possible with relative ease to transplant a fertilized human egg from the womb of its biological mother to that of a foster mother who will bring it to birth. Working women will be able to have someone else bear their babies. Childless women will be able to have the experience of giving birth to their adopted offspring. Moreover, techniques are being perfected which will permit, it is hoped, the modification of an individual's genetic inheritance. There is evidence, for example, that the action of the gene for sickle-cell anemia can be suppressed by activating or deactivating other genes to which its functioning is linked. Again, experiments have been performed indicating the possibility of making up for genetic deficiencies by implanting the needed genes. Gene therapy, chemical or surgical, thus appears to be a quite possible, if not immediate, medical procedure.

Nor do the achievements in genetics and biomedicine quite exhaust the advances being made toward the understanding of the human organism, and the possible refabrication of it. Parallel to the discoveries that I have mentioned are those in the surgery of organic transplants, the pharmacological alteration of personality, and the study of the brain and nervous system. Electromicroscopy, in the words of Sir John Eccles, "gives us a look at the components of the brain, the living nerve cells, and the connections between them, the synapses, at a level that is commensurate with their properties," and neuropharmacology "gives us an exquisite understanding of the way the synapses are working with regard to the chemical transmitters and their antagonists, so that we have the potentiality to control the operation of the nervous system in a carefully designed manner."[4]

Finally, the story cannot be complete without mention of "cloning," a process which permits an indefinite number of genetically identical beings to be produced from a single individual, without blessing of sexual fertilization. Whether the cloning of human beings will be technically feasible in the near future is a matter of dispute, but the experiment has been performed successfully with frogs, from whom no complaint has been heard. Cloning would permit people to reproduce themselves in the literal sense, to duplicate themselves genetically with exactness, a more fulfilling procedure, it must be supposed, than the messy process of ordinary procreation, which leaves so much to the random fall of the genes. Since advancing research also indicates that aging is a genetically controlled process, and that the rate of aging can be significantly slowed by diet, drugs, and genetic recoding, a new prospect opens: a world populated by centenarians in glistening health, surrounded by preselected carbon copies of themselves of assorted ages. Gone are those children with the unexpected traits that make a man or woman wonder out of what nest they came. At last we will have the young just how, and where, we want them.

III

Whatever the potentialities of biomedicine, it is easy to see why it arouses the interest that it does. The subject forces a confrontation with Good and Evil: it is like the story of Dr. Faustus, or Adam and Eve's encounter, all over again, with the Tree of Knowledge. For it implicitly asks, what shall the human species make of itself? And in asking that question it exposes our ultimate convictions.

Most important technological innovations, to be sure, raise the same question about the designs of the human species on or for itself. As C. S. Lewis once observed, in discussing technology's so-called conquest of nature, "In every victory, besides being the general who triumphs [man] is also the prisoner who follows the triumphal car."[5] Even technological innovations that do not involve direct probings inside the human body produce changes in human thinking, feeling, and conduct. They present us with new options or enhance our powers to achieve old goals, but they also foreclose options, change our goals, reduce our powers. Technology, in general, is not only an extension of human power over nature but an experiment with human nature, a test of the modifiability of the human physique, mentality, and emotional equipment, and of the costs and consequences of placing new loads on them. Nevertheless, biomedicine differs in significant ways from other kinds of technology.

First of all, we have the experience of the past, which suggests that, of all forms of scientific and technological innovation, medical discoveries—the circulation of the blood, anesthesia, antiseptics, malaria control, the Pill—have had the swiftest and most far-reaching effects on people's lives and moral horizons. Even if we discount by a prudent amount the significance of the last generation's achievements in biomedicine and related subjects, they still represent a considerable change in some of the basic parameters of human existence. To take a simple example, the classic discussion of the roles of heredity and environment may be turned upside down. It has always been thought that the "environmental" explanation of traits like intelligence, for example, was the more liberal, hopeful, forward-looking. But the day may not be that far away when genetic manipulations to improve intelligence will be a cheaper and more practical means to get results than environmental reforms, which have already been proved to be more difficult to bring about, and more disappointing in their consequences, than was supposed. Under such circumstances, environmentalists would be the preachers of pessimism, inegalitarianism, and allied heresies, and hereditarians would be the bearers of glad tidings.

Secondly, biomedicine involves introducing changes in the human creature different in a fundamental respect from those that have followed technological and scientific innovations in the past. People did not intend to reduce the average height of the British lower classes when they introduced the factory system, and they had no plan to change the formative experiences of adolescence when they welcomed the Model T. Biomedicine, in contrast, involves the deliberate, not incidental or inadvertent, modification of the human organism; and it involves, besides, the making of changes that will be irreversible. Rightly or wrongly, people in the past could make decisions about the introduction of technologies without thinking about the consequences. In the case of biomedicine that fine freedom is gone. Its various techniques may be widely adopted, and the consideration of consequences may be minimal, but the process will involve a conscious and deliberate refusal to think. Biomedicine has eliminated the insouciance with which most people have embraced technological progress. It forces consideration not simply of techniques and instrumentalities but of ends and purposes.

IV

It is, therefore, a disorienting science. The reactions to it have been like the reactions of the contemporary American mind to other disorienting events. There have been calls for additional research; interdisciplinary teams and public commissions have been created; objurgations on the guiltiness of a nation that knows no limits have multiplied; and evangelistic utterances that at last renewal has come, and the greening of America, or of all mankind, may be at hand, have also been heard.

The evangelisms have a familiar sound. On the back of Amitai Etzioni's *Genetic Fix* there is a blurb written by Betty Friedan. Mr. Etzioni, in the book, approaches the social and moral problems of biomedicine with finickiness, but Mrs. Friedan is less cautious: "Beyond the fantastic implications of *Genetic Fix* itself, Amitai Etzioni's existential act of courage in writing this book seems to me to point the new political road we must all map for ourselves now—beyond scholarly dispassion, passive compliance, or radical rhetoric mechanically fixed to the past—to take active personal responsibility for the human future." Perhaps too much should not be read into a blurb. The words are entirely conventional. But conventional indeed they are.

They express an idea that weaves through large parts of contemporary intellectual culture, uniting B. F. Skinner's scheme for salvation through operant conditioning to Herbert Marcuse's version of Freud and Marx, and joining the programs of radical feminists with those of the theorists in international affairs who held, not so long ago, that with a proper dosage of social science plus the existential courage to use advanced machinery, Vietnam could be pushed, pulled, or pulverized into the modern world. The idea is that of a human animal wholly malleable; of differences between the old and the young, between the sexes, between nations and individuals with varying life experiences, as essentially superficial, like the dirt on a shirt collar that comes out in the wash. Society, the thought goes, entirely forms men and women. Provided only that people are willing to recognize the Good and do it—"to take active personal responsibility for the human future"—society is capable of wholly re-forming them. All that is needed, as used to be said about Vietnam, is the will. The great "breakthrough" of the last five years, I heard it flatly announced by a colleague from a department of literature at a recent university meeting, is the discovery that we are all born androgynous, and that the difference between the sexes is purely cultural—a concept which led me to wonder whether instruction in obstetrics should be transferred from the medical school to the department of sociology.

The new genetics, though it stresses heredity, has paradoxically proved to be capturable by this idea of the omnipotence of society. "Society" will simply engineer heredity. In the words of the late Hermann Muller, a Nobel laureate, programs of planned eugenics provide the opportunity to guide human evolution, to make "unlimited progress in the genetic constitution of man, to match and re-enforce his cultural progress and, reciprocally, to be re-enforced by it, in a perhaps neverending succession."[6] Such hopes justify a certain impatience in the methods used to achieve them. With the harshness of a Lenin or Trotsky, Hermann Muller complained, for example, about the carelessness with which society allows people to procreate freely, and then deals with the unhappy consequences by therapy, surgery, or the abortion of defective fetuses. Soft methods such as these, in his opinion, were "a calumny on the rationality of the human race. It would be like supposing that in some technically advanced society elaborate superhighways were constructed to avoid defiling hallowed domains reserved in perpetuity for their millions of sacred cows."[7] Another Nobel laureate, Linus Pauling, not much more merciful to sacred cows, has recommended that people diagnosed as carriers of genes associated with serious diseases like sickle-cell anemia be prevented from marrying and be conspicuously marked so that they will be warned against falling in love.[8]

To be sure, Professor Pauling gives no guidance about what to do if, in this corrupt age, such people have children without marrying, or, though one hates to contemplate the possibility, without even falling in love. Nor does he discuss in detail the complications that would follow from the adoption of his proposal in a society guaranteeing certain basic liberties to all, regardless of their hereditary category. Nevertheless, such ideas should not be dismissed out of hand as so obviously simpleminded as not to be taken seriously. Simplemindedness is not a handicap in the competition of social ideas, and although the explicit supporters of an idea like Professor Pauling's may be few, the assumptions that produce it are widely prevalent.

There are mounting signs that the eugenicists' dream of a remade human breed, so long in disgrace in consequence of Nazi forays into the field, may be on its way to a comeback. (It has never, in fact, quite died. A few hundred compulsory sterilizations are performed each year in the United States, and about half the states still have compulsory sterilization laws, although they have not been actively enforced.[9]) In 1969 the legislature of liberal Oregon passed a law providing for a "State Board of Social Protection" to administer a sterilization program. The federal government is empowered under law to pay for the sterilization of minors—under certain conditions without the consent of their parents. And public discussion, on TV and elsewhere, of the desirability of sterilizing women on welfare increases. The notion has become respectable. Indeed, existing practices provide a setting in which the idea of broad eugenic planning may seem hardly more than an extension of what is known and accepted. We endorse compulsory vaccination and chest X-rays for school children. Why not mass genetic screening or other methods for avoiding the transmission of hereditary defects or for accomplishing the improvement of the human stock?

A host of gathering trends in our society favors this easy transition: the pressures for population control; the declining death rate; the growing costs of supporting the old, the sick, and the handicapped; the size of the welfare population and the resentments caused by its existence; the altered standards regarding abortion; the movements in law and morals which, with accelerating force over the last generation, have facilitated the decline of the family and of the marital idea. And to these must be added the growing disappointment or cynicism about the possibility of social improvement through institutional reform. On the Right, people can look with sympathy on eugenics, envisaging the program's being tried on others, not on themselves. And on the Left, biomedicine speaks to the hope, ever rising from the ashes, that the human race can still be made over by proper planning.

V

There are others who have responded to biomedicine with the view that it hasn't changed anything at all except man's chance to do evil: the old moral absolutes remain as valid as ever and had better be reaffirmed. The position taken by Father Robert Drinan on the specific issue of abortion is typical of the reactions of traditional moral absolutists to the more sweeping issues raised by biomedicine:

> The integrity, the untouchableness, the inviolability of every human life by any other human being has been the cardinal principle and the centerpiece of the legal institutions of the English-speaking world and, to a large extent, of every system of law devised by man..., It will be a tragedy beyond description for America if the question of legislation on abortion is resolved on sentiment, utilitarianism, or expediency rather than on the basic ethical issue involved—the immorality of the destruction of an innocent human being carried out by other human beings for their own benefit.[10]

Rabbi Immanuel Jakobovits has been equally unbending in expressing the Orthodox Jewish view of the biomedical issue of aborting fetuses known to be seriously defective:

> Most authorities on Jewish law are agreed that physical or mental abnormalities do not in themselves compromise the title to life, whether before or after birth. Cripples and idiots, however incapacitated, enjoy the same human rights... as normal persons. Human life being infinite in value, its sanctity is bound to be entirely unaffected by the absence of any or all mental faculties or by any bodily defects: any fraction of infinity still remains infinite.[11]

Rabbi Jakobovits acknowledges that Jewish law has become a little more permissive recently, and that lenient decisions have been taken by the head of the Jerusalem Rabbinical Court. He believes, however, that these "rather isolated" developments do not change basic Jewish law as stated by the Association of Orthodox Jewish Scientists of America in 1971: "Jewish law prohibits abortion when its sole justification is to prevent the birth of a physically deformed or mentally retarded child. Abortion 'on demand' purely for the convenience of the mother or even of society is strictly prohibited and morally repugnant. . . ."

There is a less explicit, but probably even more influential, form of absolutism than that advocated in orthodox theological circles, which is espoused by a good many people who would use words like "liberal" and "progressive" to describe themselves. I do not know how large a portion of the literature on biomedicine produced in the last few years consists in the rehearsal of the fears expressed in *Brave New World,* but it must be quite large. There hovers about biomedicine the scent of ancient taboos broken, of entry into forbidden territory. It stirs to life fears that go back to the oldest myths in our civilization, and revives religious attitudes about sin, trespass, and tinkering with the delicate harmonies of the Creation that lie just below the level of consciousness even in agnostics and atheists. And so there is an impulse simply to condemn the dark powers that have brought the evil thing to be.

A few years ago it was a rare day when one heard the suggestion openly made within the university world that certain kinds of purely theoretical research should be banned. But nowadays that recommendation is made daily, without apology or obfuscation, and among the avenues of inquiry nominated for this honor biomedicine rates very high. Its emergence is among the phenomena responsible for the heating up of the hostility to technology and science, and for the reawakening of suspicion toward the basic principles of intellectual freedom and rational thought.

Biomedicine, in sum, has psychic and moral reverberations that go far beyond its immediate subject matter. On the one side, it reawakens the impulse to regulate and control, to suppress the unplanned, the random, the offbeat. On the other side, it arouses the desire to stand on the unchanging truths of the ages, and to fear and resist the play of the mind for its own sake. The discussion of biomedicine has a hidden agenda as significant as its explicit one.

VI

There are some cautionary considerations which I have found helpful in interpreting the significance of biomedicine.

Despite advances in genetics, first of all, the debate about the relative significance of heredity as against environment remains unsettled with respect to the most important human traits. Moreover, settling it is impeded by the difficulty of separating environmental from hereditary influences. Is the slow-witted child of a slow-witted mother who ignored it when it was an infant a victim of heredity or environment?

Even when we know that traits are wholly inherited, like blue eyes, or partly inherited, like height, the recent developments in genetics do not necessarily put us in a position to produce inheritable traits by plan. Most of the most interesting of these traits are "polygenic": it is the copresence of a number of genes, not any single gene, that is responsible for them. Rectifying these traits is therefore a complex matter, and runs the risk of affecting whole clusters of traits in undesired ways.

There is, in addition, a fundamental difference between "negative eugenics" and "positive eugenics." "Negative eugenics" aims only to eliminate a genetic defect. It has a definable target, and the evil it seeks to combat is reasonably unequivocal. "Positive eugenics," in contrast, aims to produce a new breed possessing, for example, "on the physical side, more robust health; on the intellectual side, keener, deeper, and more creative intelligence; on the moral side, more genuine warmth of fellow feeling and cooperative disposition; on the apperceptive side, richer appreciation and its more adequate expression." (I borrow the shopping list from Hermann Muller.) Apart from the fact that we do not know that these characteristics are primarily genetic in origin, they represent intellectual pigs in the poke.

"Keener, deeper, and more creative intelligence" covers a variety of possibilities ranging from Mozart to Napoleon; "cooperative disposition" often shows itself in warmth of fellow feeling for one group and indifference or hostility to people in others; even "robust health" has a variety of meanings: shall we aim, in our eugenics program, at heavyweight prizefighters, or at wiry, resilient little men with the power to spend long hours at their desks without falling ill? In sum, "positive eugenics" aims at gross targets, and, in practically every case, at ill-defined and incoherent ones.

Moreover, "positive eugenics" makes no sense unless it is practiced on a broad social scale. It thus involves, at the least, the use of high-pressure propaganda methods, which its devotees are likely to call "education for social responsibility," and it probably necessitates legal coercion. It has the further inconvenience of inviting people to think of themselves as stud animals.

Even in the case of "negative eugenics," a distinction has to be drawn between individual action and a general program directed at cleaning out the human gene pool. It is one thing to say that people should have the right to make an informed choice concerning whether they will have a child suffering from Tay-Sachs disease; it is quite another thing to engage in genetic counseling or other measures with a view to reducing the proportion of Tay-Sachs genes transmitted to the human gene pool by people who carry them in a recessive state. The latter is surrounded by complications.

For example, some genes responsible for serious diseases are, in their recessive states, also beneficial. The gene for sickle-cell anemia appears to have been associated with heightened resistance to malaria. Further, the "dirtying" of the gene pool, as it is called, is a long-term process, for which medical progress may be expected to provide some remedies. Diabetes, a hereditary disease, is no longer commonly a lethal one. Most important of all, to speak of "undesirable" genes is to use an environment-relative term. Diabetes is a dangerous disease when diets reach a certain level of richness; it was not usually disabling for primitive hunters.

The lesson to be drawn is an old one, but it is characteristic of fashions in ideas to neglect such lessons: probably the greatest biological resource of the human species is its variety of genetic strains. Unless we can know precisely what the future environment will contain in the way of foods, germs, climate, work, and numberless other aspects of life, caution is advisable with regard to the adoption of plans for the elimination of genetic traits whose present disutility may be a passing phase.

But if the facts of genetics make the effort to recast the human species inadvisable, the facts about human desires make it doubly so. For people are probably wisest, they understand their desires best, when they are aware that they do not know what they desire human beings to be forever and ever. In time of war, the qualities sought are resilience, discipline, loyalty, physical courage; in time of peace, people praise flexibility, independence, moral courage. Assuming that we had the requisite powers, shall the moods and needs of a decade or half-decade be permitted to affect the permanent temperament of mankind?

More prickly still is the consideration that a kind of systematic doubletalk infects most descriptions of morally desirable characteristics. "He is stubborn," I say, describing behavior which, in my own case, I call "acting on principle." "Cooperativeness" is a common candidate for moral praise; still, those who cooperated with the Nazis are called "collaborators." "Initiative" is praised but not "aggressiveness," "individualism" is admired but not "egoism."

As Aristotle observed in his *Ethics,* virtues are contextually defined. An action which, in one set of circumstances, is courageous is, in another set of circumstances, foolhardy. It is the characteristic of a fully virtuous man to know when, and to what extent, to give a particular disposition or attitude its expression. Judgment and emotional imagination are the crucial ingredients in this. Anyone who has a list of simple, unambiguous moral traits by which he would define the good man reveals that he lacks precisely these qualities. Yet they are the indispensable prerequisites for planning the future.

Indeed, even if people's moral desires were more easily definable than they are, there would still be a problem. They are woefully inconstant. The hopes for the regeneration of the race nurtured by enlightened people have moved from object to object over the last fifty years—the Russian Revolution, the war in Spain, Cuba, China, psychoanalysis as a cure for politics, politics as a cure for psychoanalysis, the encounter movement, the youth movement, the black movement, the women's movement. In 1935 Hermann Muller offered Lenin and Marx as examples of the kind of people whose genetic types should be propagated. Twenty-five years later, after the Lysenko affair, he took them off the list, and the names of Einstein, Pasteur, Lincoln, and Descartes appeared on it. Despite such changes of mind, his confidence that people knew what they were doing when they planned the genetic future of mankind remained unshaken. The intellectual and spiritual peregrinations of educated people in the last half-century do not inspire confidence in any plans they may develop for the remodeling of the species. "Oh, doctor, doctor!" says Jennifer in Shaw's *The Doctor's Dilemma;* "you. . . think you are a little god. How can you be so silly?"

Finally, all of these considerations say nothing about the classic political problem of distributing burdens and benefits. Biomedicine's techniques, however refined, cannot solve this problem. Consider even the relatively simple and easy-to-define issue of eliminating recessive genes for specific diseases from the human gene pool. A hundred such diseases will shortly be diagnosable by genetic screening, and many more, presumably, after that. A very large proportion of the human beings alive, perhaps all, will be found to be carriers of this or that dangerous characteristic. Who shall submit to biological nullification and who shall not? Genetic planning introduces a new reason for human quarrels but gives us no logic for solving them.

VII

If these considerations have any merit, there are no reasons for abandoning established principles of freedom of individual choice where biomedicine is concerned. The deliberate broad-scale regulation of man's procreative life requires powers of intelligence, imagination, and emotional perspective not within the human range. The observation applies equally, I believe, to those who would redesign the human species through eugenics and those who would place absolute barriers in the way of using biomedical knowledge to alleviate individual woes. In both cases, it seems to me, people are being asked to sacrifice the direct and immediate emotions that surround the procreating and bringing up of children to an abstract idea. It is not a prudent policy or a feeling one. Beyond the point of simpler economic budgeting, the ethical-political maxim that the present generation ought to sacrifice itself for an unidentified posterity has usually led to suffering not only profound but useless. People regularly do pay attention to the future, and make sacrifices for it, but for reasons of specific affection: they care for their children and grandchildren. I am inclined to think this a surer and sounder basis for choice than the hope for a new breed or the fear that absolute moral principles will be sullied.

I may appear unfair to apply these strictures against unrestrained abstractionism to people like Father Drinan or Rabbi Jakobovits, who seem to wish only that new scientific knowledge not be permitted to tear us loose from firm and tested ethical moorings. I confess that I feel considerably more sympathy with their views, with their creature caution, their sense of knowing what they know and preferring it, than I do with any eugenic Grand Design. Yet the reactions of Father Drinan and Rabbi Jakobovits seem to me unrealistic. Positions like theirs are not likely to prevent the acceptance and widespread use of biomedical techniques; but they are likely, through their intransigence alone, to impede efforts to deal with biomedicine with prudent restraint.

And most directly related to the present point is the consideration that, like eugenicists' plans, they allow an idea to soar away from any identifiable context. "The sanctity of human life," for example, undoubtedly expresses a value, but it doesn't exist alone. The duty not to cause avoidable suffering surely also makes a claim on us. So does the duty to use limited human resources discriminatingly. This sometimes involves making distinctions among kinds of life, including, if necessary, a fetus's life from an infant's. Recognition of the plurality of human duties is not properly described by words like "sentiment," "utilitarianism," or "expediency."

I do not find persuasive the first principle Father Drinan or Rabbi Jakobovits suggests—"the immorality of the destruction of any innocent human being carried out by other human beings for their own benefit." Like all such principles it fails as a guide in all cases. How does this principle apply to just wars, for example? Does it say there are none? Or that in war there are no innocents? How does it apply to common peacetime enterprises, like coal mining or bridge building, to which civilized and decent people give support every day, and which involve the predictable deaths of some human beings for the benefit of others? Admittedly, there is always, as classic arguments maintain, the danger of "the slippery slope." It can be said that once the decision has been taken that a fetal life can be aborted because it is unwanted, we are moving down the slippery slope that will lead to the taking of innocent adult lives because they are unwanted. But there are other slippery slopes. It seems to me also arguable, and somewhat more convincingly, that when people permit otherwise avoidable suffering to take place in the name of such speculative possibilities, they are halfway down the slippery slope that leads to the righteous punishment of their fellows for the sake of an abstract creed.

The fact is that any principle has its slippery slope. One meets that danger by combining it with other principles and not allowing oneself to be guided by it alone. Thomas Aquinas, no enemy to absolute values but not a moral innocent either, observed in the *Summa* (Qu. 94) that the law of nature, "as far as general first principles are concerned," is the same for everybody, but that when we get down to particular cases "it can admit of exceptions," and is applicable unchanged "only in the majority of cases." Few people who have looked closely at the concrete situations, each different from the next, in which, let us say, the parents of predictably mongoloid children have to decide about abortion, have been capable of coming up with unbreakable rules on the matter. Catholic and Jewish clergymen, even of orthodox views, have not invariably been as uncompromising in practice as their statements in theory would lead one to expect.

As for the notion of suppressing biomedical research because it involves playing with the ultimate secrets of nature, the impulse to adopt such a view is understandable but not the ease with which some members of the intellectual world are giving in to it. That biomedicine has given mankind powers which it is capable of using for ill is evident. Technologies of extraordinary power have been turned loose in contemporary society without even the simulacrum of thought about the consequences, and now we have one more. But the research that leads to test-tube babies is also the research that leads to a better understanding of cancer. Inquiry goes where nobody can predict, and technologies are useful for good and ill. These are truths that sound tired from being repeated, but they remain true and it is sad that they so often have to be repeated. For while technology is equivocal in its consequences, one thing is not—the damage that ensues, almost always very quickly, when a field of inquiry is banned because it is said to conflict with higher moral laws. The number of subjects that can come under this ax is indefinitely large. The character of the people who have ever wielded this ax is not reassuring.

Nor is the naiveté of eugenics planners. Professor Pauling, in a society that has run into some trouble in consequence of its habit of categorizing people by race, proposes that people be visibly marked when they carry bad genes! And others from Hermann Muller down envisage the planned production of a new human breed without facing the implications for their plan of the persistence of national sovereignties. Redesigning the species is not possible except under the strongest of world governments. If it were known that the object of such a government was to make a new breed, the arguments over which present breed should be the principal model would be likely to be considerable. There would probably be words like "genocide" thrown around. This would not facilitate the attainment of such a government, which, even under present circumstances, is not precisely easy to create.

The most astonishing question of all posed by the advent of biomedicine, probably, is why adults of high intelligence and considerable education so regularly give themselves, on slight and doubtful provocation, to unbounded plans for remaking the race. The factor responsible is not biomedicine; something else can be the catalyst tomorrow. It is the larger idea which has shaped the major traumatic events of the last three hundred years of modern history. What unites the Puritan radicals, the Jacobins, the Bolsheviks, the Nazis, and the Maoists is the deliberate intention to create a "new man," to redo the human creature by design. That is the modern idea of Revolution, an idea not entertained in the ancient world except as a matter of faith, miracles, and the destruction of temporal things. It is what has lifted revolution in the modern world above purely mundane concerns like overthrowing tyranny, or putting more capable or decent people into power, and has made it a process of transcendent meaning, beyond politics or pity, and justifying any sacrifice. These are the accents with which Sir Francis Crick, still another Nobel laureate, speaks, when he states his belief that no newborn infant should be declared human until it has passed certain tests regarding its genetic endowment, and that if it fails these tests it forfeits the right to live.

The partisans of large-scale eugenics planning, the Nazis aside, have usually been people of notable humanitarian sentiments. They seem not to hear themselves. It is that other music that they hear, the music that says that there shall be nothing random in the world, nothing independent, nothing moved by its own vitality, nothing out of keeping with some Idea: even our children must be not our progeny but our creations.

Notes

1. A bill providing for the establishment of "A National Advisory Commission on Health, Science, and Society," introduced by Senator Walter Mondale, was passed unanimously by the Senate in the 92nd Congress, but failed in the House. It has been reintroduced once more in the present session of Congress.

2. For recent examples, see Amitai Etzioni, *Genetic Fix,* and Daniel Callahan, *The Tyranny of Survival,* both published by Macmillan.

3. Edgar Chasteen, "The Case for Compulsory Population Control," *Mademoiselle,* January 1970.

4. "Science and Freedom," the *Humanist,* September-October 1972.

5. *The Abolition of Man* (1965), p. 71.

6. "The Guidance of Human Evolution," in Muller, *Studies in Genetics*

(1962), p. 590.

7. "The Guidance of Human Evolution," in *Perspectives in Biology and Medicine* 3 (1959), p. 37.

8. "I have suggested that there should be tattooed on the forehead of every young person a symbol showing possession of the sickle-cell gene or whatever other similar gene, such as the gene for phenylketonuria, that he has been found to possess in single dose. If this were done, two young people carrying the same seriously defective gene in single dose would recognize this situation at first sight, and would refrain from failling in love with one another. It is my opinion that legislation along this line, compulsory testing for defective genes before marriage, and some form of public or semi-public display of this possession, should be adopted." ("Reflections on the New Biology," *UCLA Law Review* 15: 3 [1968], p. 269.)

9. See William T. Vukowich, "The Dawning of the Brave New World— Legal, Ethical, and Social Issues of Genetics," *University of Illinois Law Forum* 1971: 2 (1971).

10. "The Right to Be Born," in David F. Walbert and J. Douglas Butler, eds., *Abortion, Society, and the Law* (1973), p. 137.

11. "Jewish Views on Abortion," *ibid.*, pp. 109, 118-19.

3

Genetic Manipulation: Past, Present, Future

Darrel S. English

The Past

A smartly dressed Roman soldier anxiously paces the floor of his neatly kept modest home while his wife is attended by the family physician and midwives. With great anticipation, he imagines his firstborn child: a son who will grow with perfect god-like stature to become a Roman officer. Suddenly, there is a deafening silence followed by the cry of new life. The soldier rushes into the room for a look at his firstborn. But as he looks at the pink, squirming form, he is horrified: the child is grossly deformed, with hare lip and cleft palate. Further observation reveals other abnormalities of the head and eyes. The soldier hesitates a moment, throws back his flowing cape, draws his sword and, in one swift thrust, destroys his own creation . . .

This unpleasant scene might very well have occurred during the time of the Roman Empire. The Romans did not hesitate to purge their society of inferior-quality human beings; though they lacked any knowledge of the laws of heredity, they were aware of the hazards of passing abnormalities from one generation to the next.

Perhaps the ancient goal was to produce a race of physically perfect, god-like people. The Spartans not only practiced infanticide, but also limited the emigration of the dominant classes, imposed special taxes on the celibate, and periodically massacred large numbers of the "helots" to maintain their own social dominance over the supposedly inferior elements of the population. Chronic invalids and victims of self-indulgence were denied medical aid; the morally degenerate were simply executed.

Plato advanced the idea of race improvement in *The Republic*, with concepts similar to those of present-day stock breeders and horticulturalists. He proposed that the perfection of the race could be promoted if men and women of high quality were to unite temporarily for the specific purpose of creating superior offspring. As many people as possible were to be produced in this fashion and the children were to be raised under the watchful eyes of the state nurseries. Plato further proposed that those of inferior quality should be prevented from reproducing. If, by chance, those elements should produce children, the infants should be quickly destroyed before they had a chance to mature and perpetuate their inferiority. The end result would be a race of people with fine physical characteristics.

In Plato's Athens, where the dominant desire was to develop culturally in the arts, politics, and sciences, people of superior background were encouraged to marry and produce high-quality offspring. As Francis Galton noted, during the sixth to fourth centuries B.C. Athens produced some of the most illustrious men the world has known.

No doubt prehistoric man unknowingly practiced a crude form of eugenics, or at least physiological selection. We know from archeological discoveries that ancient man was not immune to the debilitating effects of mutations that left persons malformed. While some of these genetically maimed early humans apparently survived and were cared for by family or tribal members, most perished quickly. Competition under harsh conditions must have made survival difficult even for the healthiest. Under natural selective forces, many succumbed to the attacks of wild animals, hostile neighboring tribes, and strife within the community. Even in today's primitive cultures one finds social structures geared to the survival of the strong; the weak, the physically and mentally impaired, and the old perish.

The eugenics movement made few advances until the nineteenth century, when men like Charles Darwin, Francis Galton, and Gregor Mendel laid the groundwork for modern views on human evolvement. Their work stimulated new interest in what might have produced the present state of human achievement over the previous thousands of years, and they speculated as to what the next millenium might produce. Growing evidence in support of Darwin's theory of evolution, joined with a basic understanding of genetic phenomena, made it possible to influence and direct purposefully the evolution of domesticated plants and animals. Extrapolating from these significant successes they wondered, quite reasonably, if such procedures could be applied to the human population.

Galton, who was Darwin's cousin, led the first concentrated effort toward modern human genetic studies. He coined the term *eugenics,* which means "well born" or "true born." In his scholarly book *Enquiries into Human Faculty and Its Development,* he defined eugenics as the study of those agencies under social control that improve or impair the hereditary physical and mental qualities of future generations. He proposed that one could improve the human stock by decreasing the birthrate of unfit persons. To support his thesis, he conducted extensive studies of criminality, insanity, blindness, and numerous other detrimental human characteristics. Galton was able to identify the inheritance pattern for some traits. More significantly, he recognized the importance of twin studies as a method of determining the effects of inheritance versus environment: when the background of identical twins was comparable, the power of heredity proved to be strongly dominant over the environment. Galton's often controversial results were grounded solidly on statistical analysis of a sophistication never before achieved by biologists. More recent studies of monozygotic (identical) twins have largely confirmed his conclusions. Even when separated in early life, identical twins are remarkably similar in physical characteristics, length of life, susceptibility to disease, intelligence, and personal and social traits. (It is interesting to note that in spite of his firm convictions regarding eugenic principles, this unusually gifted man died without fathering any children of his own.)

The Present

Anxiously, a middle-aged, graying businessman paces the confines of the hospital waiting room. After several hours of chain-smoking (interspersed with nail-biting) the entrance of a white-garbed physician startles the haggard man. The broad smile on the doctor's face immediately tells the new father that all is well with his wife and new son. . .

This may not sound unusual, but it depicts one of the most remarkable events of 1974. The couple involved were unable to have children by normal means. The woman had deformed oviducts and the eggs she produced were unable to reach the area of the uterus; thus it was impossible for sperm to contact the egg and fertilize it. Similar problems render numerous women sterile— but in this case a solution was found in a laboratory in England.

Eggs were removed from the woman by laparscopy (a thin tube is inserted into the abdomen) and fertilized by the man's sperm in a sterile test tube under the watchful eyes of research biologists. One of these tiny blobs of dividing protoplasm, called a blastocyst, was then reimplanted into the woman's otherwise sterile reproductive system. Then occurred what should never have (physically) happened: the blastocyst grew, thrived, and after nine months of confinement made its second trip into the hostile environment outside the protective surroundings of the womb. The first "test tube conception" was a reality, a conception without the aid of sexual intercourse or fertilization within the female reproductive tract.

Reproductive biology has come a long way in the past several years. Medical science had been working toward this goal since 1962, when two South African ewes gave birth to lambs whose real parents resided in England. Weeks before, researchers had injected a female sheep with the follicle-stimulating hormone (FSH) and the animal had superovulated, i.e., she had been induced to shed many more than the normal one egg. The eggs were carefully collected, artificially fertilized, and implanted into the oviducts of a rabbit. This host animal, which acted as a living incubator, was flown to South Africa. There a second team of biologists removed the developing embryos and implanted them into surrogate ewes; months later lambs were born.

Transplantation of zygotes (zygote adoption) is now becoming commercially important in the improvement of domesticated livestock. Superior zygotes are flushed from the uteri of cows and transported to ranchers who are trying to improve the quality of their stock. In one generation a herd can be transformed from one of mediocre genetic constitution into a superior crossbreed of the rancher's choice. This process represents the converse of artificial insemination, which enables a prize bull to father more than 50,000 offspring per year.

Although the above procedures have been developed, their potential for bettering the quality of the human race may not be realized in the immediate future. The upgrading of the human gene pool can be divided into two genetic thrusts: negative (or preventive) eugenics, and positive (or progressive) eugenics. Negative eugenics is concerned with the elimination of genes that produce undesirable characteristics while positive eugenics is involved with the encouragement and further increase of the frequencies of desirable genes. The two branches of eugenics are identical in a real sense, because to discourage the production of deleterious traits is, ipso facto, to encourage an increased gene frequency for the desirable ones.

In the past, negative eugenics has led to sterilization and isolation in institutions. Generally, the impact of this approach has not been significant. Furthermore, to determine what constitutes an "undesirable" phenotype (particular genetic occurrence) has been a major problem; the practice of negative eugenics has not always been lawful, nor has it been ethically or morally acceptable to the majority of the population. One need only to be reminded of the three black Alabama girls who were recently sterilized on the grounds of being mentally retarded.

There exist more practical methods of negative eugenics: voluntary sterilization; medically induced abortion; general education concerning the basic laws of inheritance of lethal genes, metabolic diseases, and chromosomal aberrations; the use of birth control methods; and a general change in attitudes with regard to the desirability of small families. All of these efforts are designed to reduce the dysgenic (deteriorating) effect of perpetuating specific undesirable traits. Genetic defects may generally be classified into one of two categories. First, there are point mutations, which take place at the biochemical level and involve submicroscopic changes in the DNA molecule. Most genetic defects result from single gene mutations within the DNA molecule; the altered information that reaches the metabolic machinery of the cell is expressed as a disease. The second type of mutation is a chromosomal mutation—that is, changes within the chromosome itself (additions, deficiencies, inversions, or translocations) or variations in the number and type of chromosomes. In general, any alteration in the chromosomal makeup of the human organism results in an abnormal or lethal phenotypic expression.

The inheritance of certain genetic defects is sex-linked because the genes that determine those characteristics are located on the sex chromosomes. In human beings, one of the 23 pairs of chromosomes determines sex. If the two chromosomes in this pair are identical (XX), the individual will be female; if they are different (XY), male. Since the male derives his only X chromosome from his mother, all X-linked genes in men are maternally inherited. In females, however, the X-linked genes are derived from both parents. Thus, if a man inherits an X-linked gene for an abnormal characteristic, the characteristic is always expressed in his phenotype; whereas a woman who is only a heterozygous carrier will show no signs of abnormality.

A well known sex-linked recessive mutation is the "bleeder's disease," hemophilia. The dominant gene H which produces normal clotting factors has been altered to a recessive condition, h, and no longer has the capacity to clot the blood. Females who possess two X chromosomes may be perfectly normal genetically (HH), or they may be carriers of the disease (Hh). It is rare to find a woman with the homozygous recessive phenotype (hh). Males, on the other hand, will express either the dominant trait (H) or the recessive trait (h) since they possess only one X chromosome. Hemophilia is found in approximately one in every 10,000 male births. Defective genes like those that cause hemophilia tend to eliminate themselves from the population naturally before the defect can be perpetuated in the next generation; however, those with the gene in the heterozygous state tend to survive. Until recently, hemophilia nearly always had severe and often lethal effects. With the development of antihemophiliac sera, the effect has been greatly reduced and hemophiliacs can expect to lead normal lives and reach a reproductive age.

Phenylketonuria (PKU)—in which the child is unable to produce specific enzymes for the breakdown of one of the amino acids, phenylalanine—is a point mutation that leads to severe physical and mental impairment. Although the frequency of this defect is only 1 in 10,000, the results are devastating: soon after birth, brain cells are suffocated by metabolic by-products, and the result is severe mental retardation. Fortunately, medical science has developed a simple test that enables the physician to detect this problem soon after birth. Once diagnosed, the infant can be given a synthetic diet called lofenalac, which is low in phenylalanine. After approximately eight years, the child outgrows the potential damage to the brain and can lead a perfectly normal life even though high concentrations of the by-products remain in his system. A PKU woman who survives to reach adulthood and becomes pregnant herself must once again go on the phenylalanine-free diet. The excess by-products in her bloodstream would otherwise be absorbed by her fetus, which would suffer brain damage. A similar situation applies in the case of galactosemia or milk poisoning, where autosomal recessive mutations combine resulting in the inability to produce the enzymes necessary for the breakdown of the milk sugar galactose.

In most cases, a defective or missing enzyme is the cause of metabolic diseases. Previous attempts at enzyme-injection therapy have failed because the enzymes were not pure enough or were unable to cross the "blood brain barrier," a screening mechanism that keeps foreign material from entering the central nervous system. Advancements in this technique have been made, however, in treating Fabry's disease, an inherited, sex-linked malady. As a boy with this condition approaches his teens, he develops severe pains in his arms and legs; he dies in early middle age from kidney poisoning. In the United States approximately 150 men suffer from this rare disease. In 1967 it was found to be caused by a faulty fat-metabolizing enzyme, alpha galactosidase: because of the malfunctioning of this enzyme, fats are not broken down and accumulate in the bloodstream. Scientists at the National Institute of Neurological Disease and Strokes purified the enzyme in 1973 and injected it into a patient with Fabry's disease. They found that fat transport through the bloodstream to the kidneys was significantly reduced; the disease is thus slowed but not cured. Such experiments offer hope that a cure will be found for genetic diseases through enzyme-injection therapy.

The chromosomal mutations are of equal concern to both geneticist and physician. Normally, humans have 23 pairs of chromosomes. Occasionally a mistake in the formation of sex cells results in additions or deletions of chromosomes; moreover, a piece of a chromosome can be lost because of contact with certain chemicals such as LSD or high energy radiation, i.e. X-rays. These alterations manifest themselves in impaired development and aberrant offspring. Occasionally there is an extra chromosome—for example in the disease known as Down's syndrome, or trisomy-21, the victim has 47 chromosomes, the twenty-first being in excess. Such mutations have appeared at a frequency of approximately 1 per 650 births, with occurrence seemingly related to the age and past health of the mother. Sometimes the extra chromosome becomes attached to another chromosome and is inherited with a frequency of one in every three births for a particular mother. The symptoms of Down's syndrome include retarded growth, a fold in the eyelid (hence the old term "mongolism"), changes in dermatoglyphics, an increased susceptibility to leukemia, and mental retardation. The victims often die in their early teens from other health-related complications. There is no known cure.

Recently, much publicity has been given to the problem of the extra Y chromosome. Few laymen realize that in approximately one in every 400 live male births the XYY syndrome emerges, making it probably the most common chromosomal disorder known to man. These individuals show a wide variety of characteristics, but, to generalize, they are often tall (averaging 73.1 inches, compared to 67 inches for the normal XY individual) and suffer from acne. XYY has been found in men who have a predisposition for antisocial behavior, subnormal mentality, and even violent crime. In 1960, the XYY syndrome came to the public's attention when Richard Speck murdered eight nurses in a Chicago apartment. A routine check of his chromosomes uncovered the XYY make-up. Recent studies show that this violent nature does not invariably result from possessing an XYY complement of chromosomes; many men with XYY combinations lead normal lives. One theory attributes antisocial behavior in some XYYs to environmental factors: being taller and duller than their peers, they were taunted and teased, and so they developed aggressive behavior patterns to compensate. The point is that, although there is a correlation between XYY chromosomal structure and antisocial behavior, there may be two equally efficacious corrective techniques (psychiatric and eugenic) with very different social and political implications.

The loss of genetic material likewise results in abnormal development. Turner's syndrome occurs when one X chromosome is missing. The resulting XO female, with 45 chromosomes, is mentally retarded, short of stature, and often sterile because of rudimentary ovarian development; she frequently displays a peculiar "webbing" of the neck. One does not have to lose an entire chromosome to be affected: in humans, a loss of a small portion of the short arm of the 5th chromosome produces the Cri du chat, or "cry of the cat," syndrome. Severe mental retardation and abnormal larynx development result in a meowing cry early in childhood.

In all of these cases, an alteration in the individual's genetic makeup brings about an undesirable condition. Medical scientists are continually developing new techniques and procedures to alleviate genetic disorders: the growing field of "euphenics" is dedicated to the relief and improvement of physiological conditions that have their basis in genetic defects. Because of scientific advancements, children with phenylketonuria, galactosemia or hemophilia who receive proper treatment can now expect to live normal lives; but other disorders such as Down's syndrome, Huntington's chorea and sickle cell anemia still have no simple cure.

Fortunately, there are tests that can warn prospective parents of their potential for producing a defective child. Tay-Sachs disease is common only among Ashkenazic Jews. Parents who are heterozygous for this recessive gene may produce a homozygous defective child. The gene in question fails to produce an enzyme, hexosaminidase A, which is needed for processing fatty compounds. The accumulation of fatty materials around nerve cells causes eventual loss of motor control, mental retardation and death. At present, a simple blood test can alert parents to this danger. Similarly, sickle cell anemia, which evolved as a functional protection against malaria, is common among blacks but rare in other racial groups. In the heterozygous state (Ss), the carriers of sickle cell anemia rarely show any harmful symptoms, but in the homozygous condition (ss) the disease causes abnormal red blood cell formation, anemia, leg sores and severe pain in the joints and abdomen; early death often results. An inexpensive, painless blood test detects carriers who produce two major types of hemoglobin instead of one. Once detected, the heterozygous carrier can be counseled as to the probability of producing defective offspring.

A technique known as amniocentesis now offers a means of detecting enzymatic and chromosomal mistakes early in pregnancy. As early as the twelfth week of pregnancy, a slender needle is inserted through the woman's abdomen into the amniotic sac of the fetus. The small sample of fluid that is removed contains cells sloughed off from the skin of the fetus. These cells can be cultured and analyzed for the absence of vital enzymes, as in the case of Tay-Sachs disease, or the appearance of abnormal chromosome numbers or shapes. Liberalized abortion laws now permit parents of an abnormal fetus the option of terminating the pregnancy by therapeutic abortion. Amniocentesis is not aimed at the destruction of life but at the preservation and maintenance of a higher quality of life. For example, in a high-risk situation amniocentesis may show the fetus to be grossly abnormal and termination of the pregnancy may be the logical choice of the parents. If under the same circumstances tests show a problem does not exist, the fetal life is saved.

Still newer methods of investigation should make possible the detection of fetal defects much earlier in life. Trophoblastic cells that break away from the fetal placenta can be detected in the mother's bloodstream. These cells can be isolated and the genetic makeup of the embryo analyzed as early as the fifth week of pregnancy. Once perfected, this test will have many advantages over amniocentesis.

No one would deny the benefits mankind has enjoyed from these euphenic measures. Medical science is dedicated to the concept of lessening suffering from all types of affliction. With regard to genetic diseases, however, the population geneticist might evaluate the "state of the art" more pessimistically than would the physician. The symptoms may be treatable, but the genes that were the cause of the malady have not been eliminated. Only a few decades ago defective genes were systematically culled from the population by natural selective forces, but now more and more people with abnormal genotypes reach the age of reproduction. This has added to our genetic load and, from an evolutionary point of view, will continue to weaken the human gene pool. Therefore, the real problem has not been solved, but in fact is being complicated for future generations who will have to depend more and more on surgery, drugs, and medical care. Not that our problems could be solved by eliminating all of the defective genotypes: many normal people carry defective genes but are leading productive lives. Mutations continually recur in the population: even if it were possible to start out with a clean "genetic slate" our record would occasionally be marred by a spontaneous mutation. It is estimated that each of us, on the average, carries from four to eight defective genes. If any one of these were to combine with a similar gene from a mate, a conception would result without full genetic faculties. In other words, each conception involves some risk of producing an offspring with serious abnormalities.

Positive eugenics, aimed at producing people with presumed superior genotypes, is also plagued with many technical, legal, and ethical problems. It has long been an accepted practice in plant and animal breeding, but only scattered proponents have urged its application to human culture. Eugenics came into disrepute when Hitler's very narrow eugenic concept was implemented in Nazi Germany. Undoubtedly influenced by the distorted interpretations that certain politicians and military men had given to Darwinism, Hitler translated the clichés of "might makes right" and "survival of the fittest" into his plan of achieving a "master race." Hitler envisioned a pure stock of "Aryans"—fair, supple Nordics free from any trace of Latin or Slavic blood, to say nothing of Jewish or non-Caucasian ancestry. Hitler went so far as to consider any "Aryan" who "mixed" with a "non-Aryan" to be contaminated for life and unfit to produce acceptable offspring. Hitler's racial ideology led him to attempt the genocide of the "degenerate" Jews. His policies severely damaged the reputation of eugenics among the general public.

Unfortunately, many characteristics that we might consider desirable—high intelligence, good disposition, longevity, etc.—are not produced by a single genetic factor. They are under the direction of a complex of genes that interact with the environment in a very complicated manner to produce a given phenotype. Herman J. Müller and James F. Crow have pointed out that such traits as high IQ, longevity, and perhaps even psychic ability have not been genetically selected with any effort in the past. They postulate, however, that if selection for such traits were to be pursued, the population involved would respond rapidly and with significant results. The technological and sociopolitical means of implementing such a selection program remain problematic. Selection schemes would probably follow the lines of cattle breeding; although they might prove to be extremely successful, they might be completely intolerable from a social, ethical, and political viewpoint.

During the early 1960s Müller vigorously advocated the use of sperm banks as a means of preserving the most desirable characteristics in the human gene pool. He was deeply concerned about his Nobel Prize-winning work in the area of X-ray mutagenesis. Knowing that high energy radiation could produce mutations, and that most mutations were harmful, he feared the effects on the population of centuries of exposure to ionizing radiation. He proposed that sperm banks be set up to preserve (for later use) the best germplasm of the human population. These frozen semen samples could also be used in case of male sterility or male genetic imperfections: they would allow a couple to choose semen of men with outstanding qualities for purposes of artificial insemination. This method, called germinal choice (eutelegenesis), would ensure offpsring having desirable genetic makeup. Complete information about the donor's psychological, physical, mental, and genetic background could be provided to ensure the best possible combination of genes. It would even be possible to incorporate the genotypes of exceptional donors who had died years ago.

Artificial insemination has long been practiced in the dairy industry, enabling, for example, a prize bull to father more than 50,000 offspring in a single year. Bull sperm has been frozen for more than twelve years without undergoing any detectable genetic damage or more than a slight loss of vitality. If applied to humans, such "preadoptive" methods offer sterile men (or carriers of detrimental genes) a way to have a family of normal children. This technique is beginning to gain acceptance: an estimated 25,000 conceptions by artificial insemination occur annually in the United States. Frozen human semen has been successfully used after a year without any apparent problems. It has been suggested that these techniques would be useful for astronauts who, on long space voyages, run the risk of exposure to abnormally high amounts of radiation. By "banking" their semen for future use, they could avoid possible genetic damage; they could even have their families started during their absence.

It would be equally desirable to be able to store undamaged eggs for long periods of time. At present, no effective technique for prolonged egg preservation has been developed. By lowering the temperature of sheep eggs to 8-10° Centigrade, researchers have been successful in maintaining them up to seventy-two hours. But freezing mammalian eggs forms tiny ice crystals in the cytoplasm, thus disrupting, and even destroying, the integrity of the cell. New methods are being developed, however: it is possible to freeze mice embryos, which are subsequently thawed and implanted into a foster mother who gives birth to them. Thus both husband and wife may someday have their embryonic children placed in cold storage while they voyage in space. This practice would eliminate possible radiation damage from deep outer space; moreover, if the parents were late in coming back, the embryos could be thawed and started in an artificial womb.

More controversial than "sperm banks" or even "embryo banks" is the possibility of producing carbon copies of humans. Since the 1920s scientists have been able to grow pieces of animal or human tissue in growth chambers for indefinite periods. (The HeLa cell culture, for example, was derived from a cervical carcinoma.) These cells have survived long after the donor's death—living in culture flasks, these and similar cells repeatedly divide to produce a population of identical cells called a clone.

In the 1950s, Briggs and King demonstrated that it was possible to take the nuclei from cells in a developing frog embryo and transplant them into enucleated eggs. These eggs, with their new diploid nuclei, responded by dividing repeatedly and produced a number of tadpoles and frogs identical in genetic makeup (since the nuclei were taken from the same animal). Similar experiments were conducted by Gurdon in the 1960s with the African clawed toad, *Xenopus laevis*. Nuclei were taken from intestinal cells and cloned. Serial transplants enabled these investigators to produce many identical copies of a single nuclear type. It would seem that endless copies could be made from a single organism.

The cloning of a human being is still in the future. The frog egg, vastly larger than the human ovum, is much easier to handle technically: H. J. Müller calculated that all of the human eggs from the total population of the earth would occupy less than a gallon of space. The frog egg also comes complete with all the nutrient requirements for independent development, whereas the human egg must be implanted in the uterine wall after fertilization to permit nourishment from the placental association.

What possible value would be derived from cloning? In animal husbandry and horticulture, new strains of cereal crops and genetically pure lines of champion livestock could be mass-produced without risking the loss of desirable characteristics during the recombination of genes occurring from the normal sexual process. We might discover how to save species of wild life currently threatened with extinction. More theoretically, test-tube fertilization and cloning would increase our knowledge of human reproduction, an area in which there is much to learn; in the process, newer and more effective means of birth control might be found. Already women with infertility problems have been helped to conceive. It is unlikely that cloning and test-tube babies will usurp the traditional baby-making process for the bulk of society. But the option may exist for those who wish to choose it: Joshua Lederberg, Nobel Prize geneticist at Stanford University, has predicted that within ten or fifteen years it may be possible to use human adult skin cells to completely bypass sexual intercourse and produce a clonal human race—identical twins of the progenitors, except they will be twenty to forty years younger. Experiments with the "artificial womb" complement this research. Now that a fertilized ovum can be implanted into the womb, the way is open to "proxy mothers," who could receive the ovum of another woman, as well as a completely mechanical womb. Although the prototype of such devices has been constructed, tremendous technical obstacles remain. For example, the placenta's chief functions—supplying nourishment to the growing fetus and removing wastes—have not yet been satisfactorily mechanized. Lamb fetuses have been kept alive for several days by connecting the umbilical cord to machines that contained an artificial lung and supplied the required nutrients, but eventually the fetuses died of cardiac arrest. There would be some definite advantages to ex utero gestation devices. Basic information concerning growth and development could be more easily monitored. The new field of "fetology" could save babies who might otherwise succumb to the trauma of birth, manipulate fetal development to correct abnormalities, and change sex, size, or other physical characteristics. More than 25,000 premature babies die every year in this country from hyaline membrane disease. The artificial womb would make the possibility of a full-term ectogenic pregnancy more likely.

Artificial insemination, artificial inovulation, test-tube fertilization and artificial wombs may seem far-fetched ideas today. But only a few short years ago most people considered birth control an experiment which would never affect the masses. For some people "the pill" has already taken the fear of pregnancy out of sexual union; the next step may well be a total divorce between sex and procreation.

Considering the rising survival rates of the newborn, and the expanded life spans of the elderly, the most pressing future problem may be population. With the new reproductive control techniques, we may in the future be able to contain the world population problem through simple, universally available contraceptives. Experimental programs are testing a slowly dissolving contraceptive device, effective for several years at a time. If such long-lasting contraceptives become a reality, women will no longer have to worry about "forgetting to take the Pill."

In the near future, the techniques of frozen semen, egg storage and test-tube fertilization may be combined into an effective birth control procedure. After reaching puberty, girls could be given a thorough physical examination by the family physician, who would inject them with hormones to induce superovulation. The eggs would be collected and placed in a deep freeze; the girl would then be given a simple operation to tie her Fallopian tubes. (Such operations are already performed.) A similar procedure could be followed for each boy: semen would be collected, frozen, and labeled for future use. If sometime later the two individuals met, fell in love, and married and decided to have children, they would visit their "gene bank." If only the male had been sterilized, a simple artificial insemination procedure would be required; if the female were sterile, an egg could be "thawed" and reimplanted for normal intercourse. Assuming both partners were sterile, the egg could be fertilized in the test tube and implanted in the wife's womb.

The benefits of such a system are many, the disadvantages, few. The transient side effects and unknown long-range dangers of the Pill and IUD would be bypassed. The tragedy of unwanted pregnancy would be eliminated. (State health department surveys indicate that as many as one out of every six girls between the ages of thirteen and nineteen is unmarried and pregnant.) One can only guess how these procedures would affect our society's structure, family unit, and moral standards. Jesuit theologian Thomas Wasserman sees drastic population control as morally acceptable if necessary—and indeed, it may be as necessary as arms limitation— but he expresses an aversion, as would most people, to governmental control. Ashley Montagu and other sociologists argue that the Pill ranks among the dozen or so major revolutions in human history. Future reproductive technologies will force us to examine even more closely the role of men and women in our changing world.

The Future

An attractive young couple waits anxiously in the comfortable surroundings of General Hospital's Reproductive Engineering Wing. The man comes from a long line of genetically superior people endowed with unusual telepathic capabilities. Back in the 1960s, his ancestors discovered that pregnant women, placed in a special decompression chamber which increased the flow of oxygen to the fetus, gave birth to super-intelligent children. Many of his ancestors thus developed into articulate conversationalists by twelve or eighteen months of age. Since then, his family selected a rare set of gene mutations for the ability to communicate without speech. The woman, a tall 309-year-old beauty, is equally remarkable: her family speciality is longevity. Again, selection was the major contributing factor in this unique family line. Both families practiced the customary method of having sperm and eggs stored in the "Bank of the Future." Unique combinations of eggs and sperm formed embryos which were then placed in the "deep freeze" until it was certain that no abnormalities developed. After a certain time "on ice," the embryos were allowed to thaw out and were implanted in surrogate mothers of unusual pregnancy powers. These procedures have been a standard practice for the past several decades but this couple is the first to be involved in a new, more innovative procedure using the technique of gene analysis. Each parent supplied a few cells to be cultured and analyzed. A computer print-out was obtained for the distinctive chemical makeup of DNA for each of their genes. Instead of waiting for the right combination of genes to unite by chance, as is the usual process in sexual union of gametes, reproductive biochemists synthesized the most desired gene types from each partner. The artificially produced genes were combined into the normal set of twenty-three pairs of chromosomes, and a zygote was synthesized de novo.

The doors of the "Womb Room" open: the doctor, greeting the couple with great exultation, leads them into the nursery for their first glimpse of their eight new babies. The zygote was allowed to divide three times before each cell was separated and cloned into a new individual. Furthermore, a little fetological surgery and hormone therapy changed the sex of four of the developing embryos: the first set of opposite sex genetically identical octuplets is born. . .

Our account has gone over the brink into science fiction—or has it? Since the discovery of the nature of the DNA molecule some twenty years ago, rapid progress has been made in understanding the function of chemical transmitters of inheritance. Early in the 1960s, Kornberg and his associates synthesized DNA that was biologically active. The implications of this experiment are profound: if one can make an artificial DNA in the test tube, then perhaps someday one can create specific genes to insert into deficient cells. Microbial geneticists have known that this was possible for some time. Purified DNA from one strain of bacteria can be absorbed by another strain and integrated into the recipient cells, resulting in a change in some of their genetic characteristics, a phenomena called "transformation." In another commonly practiced technique, "transduction," viruses are used to transfer the genetic material in one bacterial cell to another. One day viruses may be routinely used to correct genetic diseases at the source of the problem: the DNA level. Genetic engineering or "algeny" would then effect a permanent cure, to the benefit of all future generations. For example, it is well known that galactosemia results from a homozygous mutant for the enzyme that breaks this sugar down. If a normal gene could be inserted for the missing enzyme, the cells could then metabolize the substrate molecules. In 1971 molecular biologist Carl Merril and his colleagues at the National Institute of Health successfully transplanted a bacterial gene for galactose metabolism into human tissue culture cells that came from a victim of galactosemia. The transduced cell appeared to be synthesizing the missing enzyme, and cell generations later the DNA substitute continues to undergo replication and transcription. The ability of a human cell to use a bacterial gene further illustrates the universality of the coding mechanism in a variety of living forms.

In 1974 this process was reversed. Animal genes were trans planted into bacteria, forming DNA "chimeras"—molecules consisting of genes from different sources. (The term *chimera* comes from Greek mythology and refers to monsters composed of incongruous parts.) Joshua Lederberg sees the technique as a major tool of genetic analysis that accomplishes at the molecular level what cross-breeding does for the whole organism. Work is currently being carried out to transform the genes responsible for making the antibiotic streptomycin from soil fungal-like bacteria into bacteria that are much easier to cultivate. The practical applications are evident: the pharmaceutical industry will have a definite economic interest in these chimeras, and agriculture is looking into the possibility of using the chimera transplant technique to transfer nitrogen-fixing genes from certain microbes to bacteria that normally live near the roots of cereal grains. The aim would be to provide nitrogen fertilizer, thus reducing the need for fertilizers, which have been skyrocketing in price.

Taking this one step further, Nobel Prize winner H. G. Khorana and his co-workers successfully isolated a single gene in *Eschericia coli*. The gene, controlling the cell's ability to incorporate the amino acid tyrosine into a protein, was analyzed for its chemical makeup, and is now being synthesized *de novo*. Since then they have concentrated on efforts to determine the chemical sequence in the DNA molecule that is responsible for turning the gene "on" and "off." The long-term goal is to synthesize the gene and its control signals totally to see if it will function in living cells of E. *coli*. Once that is accomplished, there is every reason to believe that geneticists will be able to synthesize specific genes and to incorporate them into more complex cells at will.

One of the major stumbling-blocks is determining how a cell switches genes "on" and "off." Developmental geneticists deal with the control of genes during the differentiation and development of single-celled zygotes as they develop into multicellular organisms. A basic question in this field is how a single cell produces a distinctly different population of cells that differentiate into specific tissues and organs. If geneticists learn how to "turn on and off" specific genes, they may be able to control genetic disease. For example, Cooley's anemia (found primarily among descendants of Mediterranean populations) results from too little hemoglobin production. Scientists hope someday to activate the defective gene and stimulate it into normal hemoglobin production. It is very possible that cancer might result from the effects of certain viruses on the regulatory processes of cell function. Thus, the cell, instead of keeping control of its normal functions, becomes a runaway. Some scientists believe that aging, too, may result from a series of genetic switches being turned on throughout life. If one could learn how to turn off these switches, or slow the process, life could be extended.

The biological revolution will not happen overnight. Some of it has already occurred; new discoveries will be made in the future. Here is a hypothetical schedule:

1970	Test tube fertilization of human egg
1971	Amoeba synthesized from spare parts
1972	Genes inserted into human cells
1973	Artificial gene synthesized
1974	Autoimplantation of a test-tube fertilization
1975	Zygote adoption between unrelated humans
1985	Choice of sex of offspring
1995	Genetic surgery—replacing defective genes
2000	Artificial placenta. Personality reconstruction
2025	Cloning of animals. Organ regeneration
2050	Control of aging. Cloned humans. Man-animal chimeras

2100   Brain-computer links. Intelligence enhancement
              Memory injection. Man-machine chimeras

Probably the most spectacular event in the field of human reproduction was the 1974 zygotic implant. There is little reason why this technique could not be carried out between unrelated subjects. It might be highly desirable if the woman was a known carrier of a harmful genetic mutant, since it would prevent her passing the defect on to her children, yet allow her to experience the emotional and psychological satisfaction of giving birth. Adoption is well established; zygotic adoption would actually be less radical socially than adopting a baby from an unknown source.

Amniocentesis has already made it possible to choose one's child's sex; however, it is expensive, uncomfortable, and comes too late in pregnancy. The separation of X- and Y-bearing sperm, coupled with artificial insemination, is the ideal method to ensure a baby of the desired sex. Other procedures involve sexing of test-tube fertilizations before reimplantation or the use of the vaginal douche to select the desired sperm types for fertilization, or sex reversal of embryos by hormone therapy. One would hope that parental choice will not be lopsided, and that the sex ratio will remain balanced.

It appears to be only a matter of time before we see genetic surgery by means of viruses and the development of artificial placentas to correct genetic defects and maintain embryos during development. So far, these methods have not been developed for human use. But who would have thought, thirty years ago, that a major portion of the United States population would be taking a pill to prevent pregnancy? We can no longer regard such predictions as "science fiction," nor can we assume that society will refuse to accept these radical practices.

Many of us prefer to think of the cloning of humans, organ culture for transplants, the control of aging, manipulation of memory, personality behavior, and the linking of man to other animals or to machines as science fiction. If achieved, these techniques will represent a new stage of scientific advancement. But with every advancement comes greater responsibility and often many disappointments. It will be up to our children and grandchildren to decide whether they want to risk the dangers in order to realize the potential of these techniques.

Some Conclusions

Few of us would want to go without the many benefits we enjoy from the advances made in the biological sciences over the last hundred years. Many of us would not be here to read this article if it were not for the life-saving effects of antibiotics like penicillin and streptomycin. Nor would we want to be without skilled surgery, life-saving technology, synthetic fibers, or fields of high-yield hybrid crops and specially bred livestock. The benefits of science have been enormous; yet suddenly man seems to be faced with problems of bioethics that he never dreamed existed. There is a growing fear that emerging technology, enabling man to manipulate his genetic and evolutionary future, may have outstripped his ability to deal with such problems on a social, legal, and ethical basis. In the winter of 1971, famed biologist J.D. Watson expressed concern before the U.S. House of Representatives that the general population knew very little about the profound implications of recent technological advances. Watson called for more public involvement in policy-making decisions concerning the role genetics will play in the future of mankind.

In 1974 a National Academy of Science committee appealed to scientists around the world for a complete moratorium on certain kinds of genetic experiments. With this unprecedented move, scientists for the first time in history have called for a voluntary restraint on their own work until international evaluations can be made. The appeal was directed at experimentation in the genetic manipulation of bacteria that might result in a synthetic andromeda strain, resistant to present antibiotics, which might cause epidemics or increase the incidence of cancer.

Gene manipulation will undoubtedly reach levels of tremendous technological sophistication, and society is sure to make use of its discoveries. It may generate new ways of producing therapeutic hormones such as insulin, and develop new strains of bacteria that can turn nitrogen in the air into plant food. As we gain a greater understanding of the biochemistry of various mental aberrations, gene therapy may be used to alter those states considered unacceptable or unproductive. "Pacification genes" may someday replace drugs and psychosurgery as tools of behavioral and social control.

These techniques open a Pandora's box; the question that must be asked is who will control the technological decisions made in the future? Numerous national and regional commissions have been set up to study the ramifications of genetic experiments. Individual scientists, not generally prone to taking a public stand on political and economic issues, are expressing their anxieties. Accurate information must be provided for the general public. Decisions that will affect all of us must not be left to the political and scientific elite who could use their knowledge to control the less powerful and less informed. How science is applied is a political and social issue; any decisions that are made must reflect the needs of all sectors of society. Scientists and the public face greater responsibilities than ever before: if mankind develops wisdom as well as intelligence we may be able to use our scientific knowledge to upgrade humanity and the world around us.

4

Genetic Tests Renounced over Possible Hazards

Victor K. McElheny

In an action rare in the history of science, prominent American biologists, including one winner of the Nobel Prize, are voluntarily renouncing for the present two types of genetic experiments that they consider could be hazardous.

The classic approach in the sciences has been to pursue a trail of scientific inquiry whereever it might lead. However, in line with a growing scientific concern about some implications of modern molecular biology, the scientists warned against "indiscriminate application" of new techniques involved in the experiments.

The scientists are announcing this action in a letter that, within the next week, will reach much of the world scientific community. They said they were taking the step because the gene-transplantation experiments might accidentally increase the resistance of some micro-organisms to drugs, or lead to the spread of some types of cancer-causing virus.

The letter is being published this week in issues of the American journal *Science* and the British journal *Nature*. The recommendations of the scientists have been endorsed, in an equally unusual action, by the Assembly of Life Sciences of the National Academy of Sciences.

The scientists request in their letter that Dr. Robert Stone, director of the National Institute of Health, the United States Government's leading medical research agency, establish an advisory committee to oversee experiments to evaluate and minimize the possible hazards and set guidelines for researchers in the field.

Dr. Stone reportedly has already written to the National Academy to ask it to establish the committee. The National Academy has scheduled a news conference in Washington this

From the *New York Times,* July 18, 1974, pp. 1, 46. © 1973/1974 by the New York Times Company. Reprinted by permission.

morning for signers of the letter to discuss their action.

Among the signers are Dr. Paul Berg of Stanford University Medical School, Dr. David Baltimore of the Massachusetts Institute of Technology, and Dr. James D. Watson, the Nobel Prize-winner who directs the Cold Spring Harbor Laboratory of Quantitative Biology on Long Island.

The "potential rather than demonstrated risk" seen by the scientists rises out of a newly developed technique for transplanting certain animal genes into single-cell bacteria. The discovery of this technique was reported in the *New York Times* on May 20, and shortly thereafter in the May issue of the *Proceedings of the National Academy of Sciences.*

The bacteria not only multiply the foreign genes, embodied in the genetic chemical called DNA, along with their own genes, but also provide an intensively studied context to observe how these foreign genes operate. The common bacterium of the human colon, Escherichia coli, is generally regarded as the organism that biologists have studied most completely.

The technique uses newly discovered enzyme proteins that act almost as surgical knives to cut DNA at precise points, and in a way that allows stretches of the stringlike, double-stranded DNA to be stitched together.

The technique also exploits the fact that bacteria like Escherichia coli contain small "satellite" rings of DNA, called "plasmids," which multiply alongside the much larger DNA ring containing most of the genes of the bacterium. Such plasmids can carry characteristics of a micro-organism such as resistance to one or more drugs.

The plasmids can be cut open with the enzymes, have genes from animals, viruses or other bacteria inserted in them, and then be stitched into a ring, which then can enter cells of Escherichia coli to multiply.

Work planned by several groups, including those of the signers of the letter, would, according to the signers, create "novel types of infectious DNA elements whose biological properties cannot be completely predicted in advance."

The signers said, "There is serious concern that some of these artificial DNA molecules could prove biologically hazardous."

Because Escherichia coli is found in the human intestinal tract, the scientists said, and because such innocuous bacteria can exchange DNA with other types, harmful to man, new DNA elements introduced into the bacteria might possibly become widely disseminated among human, bacterial, plant or animal populations with unpredictable effects.

This concern, based on a new technique, differs from the "genetic engineering" concepts, involving such futuristic ideas as producing whole armies of genetically identical human beings, or using viruses to inject missing genes into people, which biologists and the public have been discussing for the last decade.

The scientists asked others "throughout the world" to join them in "voluntarily deferring" two types of experiments.

One would involve creating new "plasmids" containing a combination of drug-resistance not found in nature, or in using plasmids to give such resistance to bacteria now lacking it.

The second class of experiments would involve attaching cancer-causing or other animal viruses to the plasmids, or to the DNA of other viruses.

The scientists said that such DNA molecules "might be more easily disseminated to bacterial populations in humans and other species and thus possibly increase the incidence of cancer and other diseases."

In addition, the scientists advised caution on experiments where animal DNA would be linked to bacterial plasmids.

The scientists urged that an international meeting be held early next year "to review scientific progress in this area and to further discuss ways to deal with the potential biohazards."

They said they realized that the risks were "potential rather than demonstrated" and that "scientifically worthwhile" research might be delayed. But they urged the delay "until attempts have been made to evaluate the hazards and some resolution of the outstanding questions has been achieved."

As publication of the letter neared, scientists searched for an exact precedent and found none. An agreement among non-German nuclear physicists in the early 1940s to cease publication about the splitting of the atom was not intended to halt work thought hazardous but to deny advantages to Nazi Germany, where the phenomenon had been discovered.

The spur to the scientists' letter came last year at the annual Gordon Conference on Nucleic Acids. After the conference, two of the participants, Dr. Maxine Singer of the National Institute of Health and Dr. Dieter Soll of Yale University, wrote a letter warning about the risks in joining DNA from "diverse sources."

That letter was published in *Science* last September 21.

A meeting to draft the current letter was held in Cambridge, Mass., in April.

Other signers included Drs. Stanley Cohen, Ronald Davis and David Hogness of Stanford University, Richard Roblin of Harvard Medical School, Norton Zinder of Rockefeller University, Daniel Nathans of Johns Hopkins University, Herbert Boyer of the University of California and Sherman Weissman of Yale University.

5

Genetic Engineering

Joseph Fletcher

Of all phases of the new molecular biology and reproductive medicine, what we call "genetic engineering" is furthest from being "operational" or in practical use. Genetic intervention in humans to eliminate inborn physical and mental defects is not here yet. But it looms ahead. Since Crick and Watson deciphered DNA's three dimension double-helix basepair structure more than twenty years ago we have already seen the nucleic acid code broken, then an active viral gene synthesized, and at the practical level the green revolution's genetic production of supercereals and miracle rice in the "hungry Third World."

Morally, genetic engineering is good when it serves human needs, both health and happiness. If genetic manipulation were not possible in agriculture and plant physiology we would be back where Stalin and Lysenko stalled Soviet biology. If we were unable to do it in animal husbandry we would have to say good-bye to the rational reproduction of meat, work and hide animals, livestock improvement, and so on. These farming and herding techniques are for human benefit, and there is no ethical cut-off point at which to clamp an arbitrary stop on the use of genetic controls for the health and quality of human beings themselves.

Two different uses are up for approval: therapeutic or medical treatment, and the *design* of genotypes preconceptively. While some people object to all genetic intervention, others only object to genetically designing human beings—not to repairing genetic faults *after* they are conceived or born. In short, they justify it for treatment but not for prevention.

This is somewhat more humane than the blanket condemnations but hardly any more rational. It is absurd to be willing to cure human ills or lacks but unwilling to avoid or supply them before they afflict us. Such a strange posture is ethical nonsense. For example, in the relatively benign area of cosmetic surgery for disfiguring physical traits, who would prefer to have it done over and over again from generation to generation when it could be obviated once and for all by genetic intervention?

Still others would condemn any use of genetic controls to produce a "strain" of men with long arms to fit them to be orchard workers, or to produce a family of people with oversize lungs for sponge fishing or pearl diving.

Ethical questions are raised about using genetic control to choose the phenotypes of *future* individuals.[1] But this is after all only another version of the ethical questions we are already facing when we reproduce with known traits. We have always had to weigh the cost of our choices and purposes against our needs, and we always will. The only change would be for the good, because we would have more control with which to do what we think is right.

A sensible policy is to breed animals for special purposes instead of humans, where possible, if the specialization delimits human capacities. Dolphins, fish, pigeons, primates are even now being used to do dull or dangerous work for us. We could even design species from scratch. There is no need to drag humans down genetically to do special or menial jobs; we can bring animals *up*, to do them. As Sir George Thompson sees it, "Very large modifications in the wild species can no doubt be made."[2] For example, animal brains can be markedly improved by doses of the twenty-first human chromosome. And rather than providing people with low IQs to do dull work we might take Shaw's advice (*The Intelligent Woman's Guide to Socialism*) and pay normal people extra high wages to do what most of us don't want to do.

Human Beings, Being Human

Human beings, in order to qualify as human, have to be something more than just biologically classifiable as organisms of the species *homo sapiens*. They have to have individual or separate existence ("viability") and they have to be actually "sapient"—that is, possessed of a functioning cerebral cortex—some minimal level of intelligence.

Therefore an individual of the species who is not yet human, a fetus, and one who has ceased to be, a "brain dead" patient, is without the status of being human or of human being. The sadness of abortion is that it means letting a potential go—but it is only a potential, not a reality; the sadness of "pulling the plug" on an irreversibly comatose patient is that it means accepting the bitter fact of a loss—acknowledging that a human being is now no more. But the point is that abortion and "brain death" terminations are *biocide,* not homicide. All talk of "killing a human being" in such cases is therefore ethically off the track.

Incidentally, the nearest thing to a specifiable "moment" for *becoming* human is when a fetus is respirated after birth—that reflexive and explosive gulp of air starting the lungs to work. This is what Plato contended. Only on his terms can it make sense to speak of the "moment" of becoming human. The "moment" of death, of *ceasing* to be human, is quite commonly unspecifiable. In any case, being human is two things essentially—intelligence and "going it alone" as an individual on one's own lungs.

Hybrids

But hold on. What if an ape had the intelligence and sensibilities of a human, and a human had only the capabilities of an ape? Which would be the human being? The answer is plain; the ape would be the human being.

This is no mere play on words. All mammals, man among them, are remarkably close biologically. Modern biology can devise "chimeras" or combinations of humans and animals, and also "cyborgs" or combinations of humans and machines. Gerald Leach warns us against the Minotaur, a mythical creature half man and half bull who was hidden away because it was too horrible to look upon.[3] The basic fact is that the body cells of all species will cross-fuse, and the germ cells of many—though not all—will unite sexually.

If a prosthetic device, perhaps an intricate mechanical hand or leg, supplies a person with 50 percent or more of the function lost in an amputation, that is morally good. An artificial kidney or hemodialysis machine is morally good. This applies equally to heart pacemakers, dacron arteries, metal bones, ceramic hipjoints. All such technical contrivances are cyborgs or man-machine "hybrids."

Man-animal combinations are in the same ethical class. If a

cow's kidney is "grown" into a patient's thigh to help cleanse his blood, after his own kidney function is gone, that is morally good. If an animal's organ or tissue is used to replace something lost by a human (an interspecific transplant) that is good. These are examples of man-animal combinations for medical purposes. And the day may come when replacement medicine will be keeping herds of animals on hand, to supply physicians with what they need. It would mean more "live" rather than transshipped cadaver transplants, and it would relieve human beings of the risks or inconveniences of the donor role.

But what of hybridization for nonmedical reasons? Chimeras or parahumans might legitimately be fashioned to do dangerous or demeaning jobs. As it is now, low grade work is shoved off on moronic and retarded individuals, the victims of uncontrolled reproduction. Should we not "program" such workers thoughtfully instead of accidentally, by means of hybridization? Cell fusion and putting human cell nuclei into animal tissue is possible (such hybrid tissue exists already as a matter of fact).

Hybrids could also be designed by sexual reproduction, as between apes and humans. If interspecific coitus is too distasteful, then laboratory fertilization and implant could do it. If women are unwilling to gestate hybrids animal females could. Actually, the artificial womb would bypass all such repugnances. In some cases even the sterility of hybrids might be overcome. (Euphenic changes, such as cell fusion tissues would be, are not transmissible genetically.)

Contrived in order to protect human beings from danger, a social reason, or from disease, a medical reason, chimeras and cyborgs would be morally justified. What counts is human need and well-being.

Notes

1. Gerald Feinberg has put it neatly. Much as we dislike making plans which restrict the freedom of future generations, we cannot escape doing so. "An inescapable result of the one-way flow of time is that we are born into a world we never made." He adds, "I do not think that any new moral principle is established" when we exercise our honest judgment about what is best for our descendants. *(The Promethean Project* [Garden City, N.Y.: Doubleday, 1969], pp. 203-5.)

2. *The Foreseeable Future* (New York: Viking, 1960), p. 98.

3. *The Biocrats* (New York: McGraw-Hill, 1970), p. 98.

6

Should Man Control
His Genetic Future?

Donald Huisingh

In recent years, many scientists have begun to emerge from the ivory towers of pure scientific research and to become actively engaged in discussions with nonscientists. The scientists are beginning to realize their ethical responsibilities and obligations. Their concern has developed most rapidly since the discovery of the awesome power of atomic energy. This event has emphasized the need for scientists to inform their fellow citizens about the findings of science and the implications they may have for their lives and those of future generations.

Today scientists are speaking to representatives from all walks of life, including politicians, theologians, economists, and laymen in general. As concrete examples, three separate symposia dealing with "Man and His Future" have been held within the last four years.[1] The speaker lists were comprised primarily of physical and biological scientists.

None of the speakers claimed to have final answers about what direction man should take in the future. Most of them indicated various alternatives and discussed the probable results, but few grappled seriously with the quandaries that are likely to result in the pursuance of any particular course.

It is not surprising that most scientists are reticent to speak about the moral and ethical considerations of their work. They have tended to relegate religion to certain discrete times and places in their lives and to do the same with their science. Thus, few have had to grapple earnestly with the fundamental moral and ethical problems their work may raise. Furthermore, more scientists (I for

From *Zygon* 4 (1969), pp. 188-199. Reprinted by permission of the author and the University of Chicago Press.

This paper was originally prepared for presentation to the Experimental Study of Science and Religion at North Carolina.

one) came through undergraduate and graduate training in the physical and biological sciences with little formal experience in the social sciences. Scientists also appreciate the necessity to specialize and are aware of the pitfalls of speaking beyond their specialty, so they have tended to shy away from the territory of the moralist and the ethicist.

I feel uncomfortable in the role I try to fulfill in this paper: to write about the "Ethical Issues of Genetic Manipulation." I am not an ethicist, nor am I primarily a genetic specialist. In what follows, however, I will first attempt to sketch briefly some of the alternatives science has made or is likely to make available to man to enable him to manipulate and direct the future of the human race. Second, I will discuss the problems involved in employing some of these alternative means and suggest tentative guidelines in their development and application.

Possible Approaches to Genetic Manipulation

There are three main categories of proposed approaches to genetic manipulation. They are. (1) euphenic engineering, (2) genetic engineering, and (3) eugenic engineering.

By *euphenic engineering,* Lederberg[2] refers to the modification or control of expression of the existing genetic information (genes) of an organism so as to lead to a desirable physical appearance (phenotype).

Genetic engineering is defined as the change of undesirable genes to more desirable forms by a process of directed mutation.

Eugenic engineering involves the selection and recombination of genes already existing in the "gene pool" of a population. The term eugenics was originally coined by Sir Francis Galton in 1883 to designate his aspiration to improve the human race by scientific breeding.[3] The word is derived from the Greek root, *eugenes,* which means "well born."

Euphenic Engineering. Euphenic engineering in its simplest forms already is common practice. For example, lack of the capacity of an individual to produce insulin results in a disorder called diabetes. The expression of this genetic abnormality can be prevented by regular injections of insulin. Similarly, normal blood constituents such as gamma globulin now are supplied routinely to individuals who do not have the genetic information to synthesize these necessary blood components. Two other genetic defects lead to mental retardation because of the accumulation of harmful metabolic products. The diseases, phenylketonuria and galactosemia, result from an individual's inability to utilize the amino acid phenylalanine and sugar galactose, respectively. These diseases do not develop if the afflicted individual's intake of these molecules is restricted by careful control of his diet.

In these examples, expression of available genetic information was manipulated so as to minimize deleterious effects. As the factors which regulate and control gene action are more thoroughly understood, it is very likely that many other types of euphenic engineering will be possible. Suggestions of what the future may hold are evident by the following examples. It has been found that an injection of the anterior pituitary growth hormone into developing rats increases their brain size by 76 percent and increased their capacity to learn by an equivalent amount. There is one report of a similar response in a human child that received an injection of this hormone in its fourth month of fetal development. There is also a report of work being done in South Africa in which pregnant women are placed in decompression chambers for varying periods of time. The children which result are said to be superior to their siblings in intellectual capabilities.

It will be only a matter of time before many additional manipulations will be feasible, especially as we learn selectively to switch on or off at will the action of desirable or undesirable genes at specified periods in a person's life. The possibility of controlling the realization of the hereditary potential of the individual is impressive.

Genetic Engineering. Genetic engineering is in its infancy in its applications to humans, but information already available suggests at least three possible approaches: (1) transduction, the virus-mediated transfer from one cell to another of genetic material; (2) transformation, the incorporation of a segment of DNA from one cell into the genetic material of another cell; (3) directed induction of mutations of specific places on the chromosomes (gene loci).

An example of transduction in humans was reported recently by Rogers of the Oak Ridge National Laboratory. He showed that the Shope virus, which causes tumors in rabbits, also induces the synthesis of a distinctive form of the enzyme arginase which lowers the concentration of the amino acid arginine in the rabbit's blood. Dr. Rogers wondered if this virus would also lower the arginine concentration in human blood. Because one may not infect human beings with animal viruses for experimental purposes, he had to get an answer to this question indirectly. He compared the blood of a number of people who had worked with, and therefore been exposed to, the Shope virus with the blood of randomly selected individuals as controls. He found that many of the researchers working with the virus were carrying "virus genetic information." They had lower arginine levels than controls and had specific antibodies against the distinctive form of arginase, indicating that the virus DNA had supplied the information for the synthesis.

The Shope virus, Rogers suggests, is a harmless "passenger" virus in these people. It is possible that there are other such viruses. Perhaps some of them carry genes that would be useful in the treatment of genetic diseases. It is conceivable that a harmless virus might even be utilized as a vector for specific information in the form of tailor-made DNA that could be attached to the virus and transferred by the process of transduction.

Szybalska of the McArdle Cancer Laboratory at the University of Wisconsin has reported that human cells in tissue culture can be transformed.[4] She found that the genetic ability to synthesize inosinic acid pyrophosphorylase could be transferred to cells that lacked this capacity by the application of DNA containing the appropriate genetic information.

Bentley Glass[5] in commenting on Szybalska's work has stated: "It may be feasible and possible in the near future to treat a germ cell defective in some gene with DNA from one known to be sound in that respect. By so doing it may be possible to improve the genetic content of the individual's reproductive cells and hopefully improve the performance of his progeny." This may be feasible, but not necessarily either advisable or wise. Within just a few years, however, we must decide whether to permit such engineering of human reproduction.

Tatum believes that "genetic engineering" by directed mutation can be seen as a possibility in humans. In microorganisms we already are learning techniques for producing mutations in a nonrandom fashion by the use of chemical mutagens such as nitrous acid and synthetic molecules related to nucleic-acid bases. These latter analogues are incorporated into DNA and upset the replicative process so as to cause the replacement of the original natural base by another one—thus producing a mutation.

Another potential approach to directed mutation is through the synthesis in the laboratory of a desired molecule of DNA. This tailored DNA molecule, if it can be isolated in pure form from an organism or cell, can probably be replicated by already known enzymatic processes to any needed quantity. This new or modified gene can then be introduced into the mammalian cell in culture as in bacterial transformation.

Eugenic Engineering. Muller very pointedly says that while genetic engineering may have some applications in the future, it will be a long time before many of the technical difficulties are removed and the methods will be applicable to a sizable segment of the population.[6] Further, he indicates that euphenic engineering, while it may be extremely beneficial to the individual, does no good for the human race as a whole. On the contrary, by keeping a genetically defective person alive and allowing him to reproduce, we are increasing the frequency of deleterious genes in the population. Muller suggests, therefore, that we ought to employ a technique which is already possible: eugenic engineering through choice of desirable germ plasm.

Immediately, the term eugenics elicits a negative response on the part of many people, because to them eugenics and racism are synonymous. To others, eugenics means voluntary or mandatory sterilization of individuals who carry certain genetic defects. This latter approach to eugenics has been termed negative eugenics. Though such responses are understandable if the negative point of view of eugenics is maintained, Muller observes that they are readily modified by sincere thinking individuals if positive eugenics and the positive point of view are considered.

What is meant by positive eugenics? Muller develops his arguments for the application of artificial insemination with selected germinal material as a technique in positive eugenics. He says, "For any group of people who have a rational attitude towards matters of reproduction, and who also have a genuine sense of their own responsibility to the next and subsequent generations, the means exist right now of achieving a much greater, speedier, and more significant genetic improvement of the population, by the use of germinal selection, than could be effected by the most sophisticated methods of treatment of the genetic material that might be available in the twenty-first century."

The idea of artificial insemination per se is not new, nor is it completely objectionable. In the United States in 1962, more than 10,000 children were "fathered" by this method.[7] In most of those cases, the husband was either sterile or was carrying some genetic defect. The seminal donors were chosen by the doctor from men with body build and other morphological features similar to the husband, so that the resulting progeny would pass as the natural offspring of the legal family. The donor's anonymity was maintained to avoid paternity suits. According to Muller, we have among such couples many who would be happy to play a role in the decision of what germinal material is to be employed. "We are thus missing a golden opportunity to begin to consciously improve the genetic complement of the human race," Muller contends. According to him, intelligent germinal choice ought to be encouraged as the most effective way of rapidly achieving evolutionary improvement of the human race. Therefore, semen banks should be established, and the husband and wife ought to be permitted to select semen from donors of highest proven physical, mental, emotional, and moral traits. In order for a sound judgment to be made of the genetic potential of an individual donor, at least twenty years should be allowed to elapse after the donor's death before the deep-frozen semen is used. The men who earn enduring esteem can thus be called upon to reappear age after age through their preserved semen.

In addition to semen banks, it will soon be possible to store human ova as well. It is already possible to fertilize the human ovum in vitro and to implant the resulting embryo into the womb of a foster mother. It may also be possible in a few years to permit the embryo to develop to "normal" maturity in artificial glass wombs.

In fact, Dr. Daniele Petrucci of Bologna, Italy, has already done extensive experimental work with human embryos in vitro. Apparently, some technical difficulties still exist, because none of the embryos have lived beyond fifty-nine days.[8] There are also theological and legal difficulties; he was told by irate church officials and local legal authorities to discontinue this type of experimentation or be tried for murder. It takes little stretch of imagination to see that soon someone somewhere will make the necessary breakthrough and it will be technically possible to develop human beings in the laboratory from the sperm and eggs of any man or woman without restriction to time or place of the donor. In this way wide numbers of individuals could be produced by genetic selection from especially able parents. Further, as euphenic engineering progresses, it will be possible to nurture the developing embryos in different types of environments and thereby condition their mental constitutions. It will not be necessary for a woman to endure the discomfort and pain of carrying a child during the prenatal period. She would, of course, not get much psychological pleasure out of visiting the laboratory where her child was developing.

Does this sound too futuristic and too much like something taken from Huxley's *Brave New World?* Many people do not think so. In fact, in September 1965, the president of the American Chemical Society, Dr. Charles C. Price of the University of Pennsylvania, urged at the society's national meeting in Atlantic City that the United States make "creation of life" in the laboratory a national goal.[9] He was speaking of creation of life *de novo* from simple inorganic and organic molecules, a feat far more complicated and difficult than merely growing an embryo to maturity in vitro.

I have tried to indicate some of the types of possibilities that are or may be feasibly applied in directing the future of man. Many questions and problems present themselves. Guidelines are needed to help the scientist choose what types of research he ought to be engaged in, to aid the technologist to select the techniques he should make available to the population at large, and to enable the politician to cope with the social, legal, and political problems which will arise as these techniques are used. With this "Biological Bomb" already about to explode, the need to face the complexity of the problem involved takes on acute, do-it-now urgency.

Problems and Guidelines

The possible approaches to genetic manipulation we have discussed raise many ethical questions, including: (1) What is the essence of human life? (2) Is the human body a sacred vessel of man's soul and spirit, or is he merely at that position in biological evolution to know that he is a part of evolution and can do something about his own future evolution? (3) What absolute human values are we eager to retain? (4) What values are only relative in a particular sociological, theological, and political framework and as such should change with future evolutionary changes? (5) What are man's biological rights and responsibilities as individuals and as members of the species *Homo sapiens?*

If we accept the possibility of improving man by germinal and oval selection, the following questions arise: (6) Are there any truly ideal genotypes? (7) What are objective criteria by which they can be selected? (8) Who singly or collectively could objectively select individuals who fulfill these criteria once they are agreed upon? Since the eugenic approach would necessarily be a long-term project, it would have to have built-in mechanisms to ensure that the goals and objectives did not change with every new generation. This would necessitate the development of breeding plans. (9) Could such plans for the population be pursued without at the same time taking away much of the freedom of the individual? (10) Should the individual's freedoms and rights be secondary to the supposed good of the human race as a whole?

Let's take a look at what might happen if we subject man to a program of planned eugenics. William Shockley in a discussion of this subject stated, "I believe the difficulty with planned eugenics is that we are forced to think of ourselves and other people as being not solely warm, living human beings with whom we can establish personal relationships, but as *objects* which can be thought of and dealt with statistically and analytically"[10] ... goes on to say, "My own reaction reminded me of a quotation expressing the same feelings in T. S. Eliot's *The Cocktail Party*":

> Nobody likes to be left with a mystery.
> But there's more to it than that. There's a loss of
>   personality;
> Or rather, you've lost touch with the person
> You thought you were. You no longer feel quite human.
> You're suddenly reduced to the status of an object—
> A living object, but no longer a person.
> It's always happening, because one is an object
> As well as a person. But we forget about it
> As quickly as we can. When you've dressed for a party
> And are going downstairs, with everything about you
> Arranged to support you in the role you have chosen,
> Then sometimes, when you come to the bottom step
> There is one step more than your feet expected
> And you come down with a jolt. Just for a moment
> You have the experience of being an object
> At the mercy of a malevolent staircase.

Or, take a surgical operation.
In consultation with the doctor and the surgeon,
In going to bed in the nursing home,
In talking to the matron, you are still the subject,
The centre of reality. But, stretched on the table,
You are a piece of furniture in a repair shop
For those who surround you, the masked actors;
All there is of you is your body
And the 'you' is withdrawn.[11]

Do we dare withdraw the "you-ness" from human beings? Do we have the option to treat man as a manipulable object or is he to be treated as an inviolable individual at the center of reality? Is there something here that we must strive to retain? Is it possible that in the process of attempting to call the shots for human evolution, one will destroy those attributes that make him human? Muller says, "No, for by selection of individual sires who have demonstrated a genuine warmth of fellow-feeling, a cooperative disposition, a depth and breadth of intellectual capacity, moral courage, an appreciation of nature and of art, a healthful, vigorous constitution, and highly developed physical tolerances and aptitudes, the progeny of such progenitors are bound to be more human, not less."[1][2]

The question of our ability to select objectively such qualities looms as a great obstacle; but the problem of finding anyone with all of these attributes in desirable proportions is even more formidable. Besides that, it is believed that everyone carries an average of four to ten recessive lethal genes which express themselves only in the homozygous condition or only in the presence of certain modifier genes or under certain environmental conditions. Even the best phenotype may have these genes lying hidden.

Let's assume, however, that we found outstanding individuals of the types desired. What is the probability of improving the heritage of the human race appreciably? To answer this, I quote from Bentley Glass's article, "Human Heredity and the Ethics of Tomorrow":

The fertilized egg contains 46 chromosomes, 23 of them inherited from the egg and 23 from the sperm. The number of different genotypes that might be present in a single fertilized egg, if there were only 23 differences between the genes in the two sets of chromosomes in the father, and 23 other differences between the genes in the two sets of chromosomes in the mother, i.e., one difference per pair of chromosomes, would be $(2^{23})^2$. That is to say, the mother could potentially produce 2^{23} or 8,388,608 genetically different sorts of eggs, and the father an equal number of sperms with different genotypes. Hence there is the possibility through random fertilization of nearly 70 trillion genotypes of offspring. That would amount to about 2,300 times the present population of the entire world. This means that the variety of human genotypes is essentially inexhaustible and that there is only an infinitesimal chance that any two persons will be identical in all genetic respects with the exception of identical twins, triplets, etc.[13]

Besides this, many of the desirable attributes of man are inherited not as single genes but as multiple genes.

Thus, even if we were capable of selecting outstanding semen and ova donors, a large degree of variability would be expected in the progeny. There would, however, be a large number of genes held in common by the offspring. Not only would it be undesirable sociologically to have large numbers of humans of very similar genotypes, but biologically it may even prove to be disastrous, because nature puts a premium on variability. Let me cite two examples of what could happen if homogeneity were achieved in a large segment of the human population.

Wheat breeders have selected, crossed, backcrossed, and selected again for desirable agronomic qualities in wheat. A few years ago, they came out with a variety which they said had tremendous genetic potential for productivity and also carried a high degree of disease resistance. In a few years, thousands of acres of America's rich wheat lands were planted with this variety of wheat. But, in 1952, a new race of wheat stem rust appeared which completely overcame the disease resistance of this variety. Two years later only a few acres of this wheat were to be found anywhere in the country. That variety of wheat was fine in the old environment but not in the new one; so too is the possibility with man. New strains of bacteria, fungi, and viruses are arising all the time. If there were a large number of people who held many genes in common, they could all rapidly succumb to a new strain of microorganism that was pathogenic against those genes.

An example from the genetics of fruit flies also is relevant here. In a certain strain the female flies have been shown to pass on through their eggs a virus which infects the developing young. This virus makes the individuals susceptible to CO_2 and has been called the CO_2 lethality virus. Similar transovarian transmission of viruses in humans is possible, and if the ova of several individuals were widely used, the likely results are obvious.

This discussion of the application of eugenics for human betterment has been based upon the following assumptions: (1) we could objectively agree what qualities to select for, (2) we could quantify and select these qualities, and (3) genetics is the most important factor in determining that an individual have or develop the desirable traits listed earlier.

Without going too deeply into the nature versus nurture argument, I would like to cite the statements of two noted authorities. Nobel laureate Dr. Francis H. C. Crick, physical biologist at Cambridge University and winner of the Nobel Prize in 1962 for his contribution to our understanding of the physical arrangement of DNA, is reported to have said, "Humans probably will not be improved or altered by genetic manipulation in the future; education and environment are more important than genetics."[14]

Dr. Bentley Glass, in a similar tone, says:

> Modern man has been on the earth for an immense stretch of time, at least 40,000 years, and maybe several hundred thousand, without much change in his skeletal anatomy. We are therefore justified, I think, in regarding all his tremendous human advance in culture and civilization, in material power and relative understanding of nature, as having occurred with little if any, genetic change. The great advances made by modern man, therefore, reflect no change in his biological heritage but represent a new phenomenon, the advent of cultural transmission, the accumulation of knowledge and its transfer from one generation to the next. Equal opportunity must be coupled with freedom of the individual if it is to lead to fullest development of the potential of the genotype.[15]

Thus two outstanding experts in the area of genetics seem to say that it is not desirable, nor is it likely to be fruitful, to involve human beings in Muller's grand genetic experiment. I concur with that conclusion. Most people never approach a realization of their genetic potential even for short periods of time because their society has not provided the educational opportunities for them to develop fully their intellectual capabilities. In additional cases the sociological mores, the political machines, and the theological institutions have erected further barriers to the individual's progress. In short, their individuality, personality, and humanity have never been developed. We ought to concentrate on maximizing the nurture of every individual so that he more nearly realizes his existing genetic potential, and move very cautiously into the area of germinal selection experiments.

Much more could be stated in summary about other possible approaches to the future of man. For example, it seems likely that negative eugenics should be continued, but it poses the ethical problem of selection of some individuals as not being fit to reproduce. In some extreme cases few people would disagree that some individuals do not have the right to reproduce because of their load of genetic defects. However, very few people would agree where the cutoff point should be.

I anticipate that genetic engineering will be found to be helpful in modifying the genetic information of individuals, but it is not likely to be a significant factor in the human population as a whole. On the other hand, progress in euphenic engineering and the provision of favorable conditions for human development and self-actualization are likely to be the most significant ways by which man will direct his own evolution. There will be many facets of the "scientific engineering" of man which will pose serious ethical problems. The politicians, lawyers, theologians, social scientists, and the general public must all be informed of the alternatives which will be available to them. They must be informed of the possible benefits and problems in order to be in a position to make intelligent use of the new tools science will provide.

What general guide will all these people use in deciding whether a particular type of research should be engaged in or whether a particular practice should be condoned and used? I would like to paraphrase what John Baillie has to say in his little book, *Natural Science and the Spiritual Life.* The future of man is secure only as long as the virtues of humility, tolerance, and impartiality are retained as absolute standards. Within this framework we should use scientific advances as tools to serve society.[16]

The time ahead is uncharted. No one has been there, so there are no experts. Each of us whose body and brain may be modified or whose descendant's characteristics may be predetermined has a vast personal stake in the outcome. We can help to insure that good will be done only by looking to it ourselves. We must be careful to retain the individuality of the individual and the personality of the person, or else the humanity of the human may be lost.

Notes

1. See J. D. Roslansky, ed., *Genetics and the Future of Man* (New York: Appleton-Century-Crofts, 1966); T. M. Sonneborn, ed., *The Control of Human Heredity and Evolution* (New York: Macmillan, 1965); and G. Wolstenholme, ed., *Man and His Future* (Boston: Little, Brown, 1963).

2. See Wolstenholme, pp. 263-73.

3. Anram Scheinfeld, *The New You and Heredity* (Philadelphia: J. B. Lippincott, 1950), p. 679.

4. Elizabeth H. Szybalska and W. Szybalska, "Genetics of Human Cell Lines. IV. DNA—Medicated Heritable Transformation of a Biochemical Trait," *Proc. Nat. Acad. Sci.* 48 (1962): 2026-34.

5. C. Stern, *Principles of Human Genetics* (San Francisco: W. H. Freeman, 1960), p. 753.

6. See Sonneborn, pp. 100-122.

7. See Wolstenholme, pp. 258-62.

8. "Control of Life. I. Exploration of Prenativity," *Life,* September 10, 1965, pp. 60-79; "Control of Life. II. Gift of Life from the Dead," *Life,* September 17, 1965, pp. 78-88; "Control of Life. III. Spare Parts for People," *Life,* September 24, 1965, pp. 66-84; and "Control of Life. IV. The New Man—What Will He Be Like?" *Life,* October 1, 1965, pp. 94-111.

9. "Control of Life. IV. The New Man—What Will He Be Like?" *Life,* October 1, 1965, p. 94.

10. See Roslansky (n. 1, above), pp. 96-97.

11. T. S. Eliot, *The Cocktail Party* (New York: Harcourt, Brace & World, 1950), pp. 29-30. Copyright 1950 by T. S. Eliot. Reprinted by permission of Harcourt, Brace & World, Inc. and Faber and Faber Ltd.

12. See Wolstenholme (n. 1, above), pp. 247-62.

13. Bentley Glass, *Science and Ethical Values* (Chapel Hill: University of North Carolina Press, 1965), p. 101.

14. "Little Change Likely," *Industrial Research* (March 1967), p. 36.

15. Bentley Glass, "The Ethical Basis of Science," *Science* 150 (1965): 1254-61.

16. John Baillie, *Natural Science and the Spiritual Life* (New York: Charles Scribner's Sons, 1952), pp. 34-43.

7

On Redoing Man

Kurt Hirschhorn

The past twenty years and, more particularly, the past five years have been an exponential growth of scientific technology. The chemical structure of the hereditary material and its language have essentially been resolved. Cells can be routinely grown in test tubes by tissue culture techniques. The exact biochemical mechanisms of many hereditary disorders have been clarified. Computer programs for genetic analysis are in common use. All of these advances and many others have inevitably led to discussions and suggestions for the modification of human heredity, both in individuals and in populations: genetic engineering.

One of the principal concerns of the pioneers in the field is the problem of the human genetic load, that is, the frequency of disadvantageous genes in the population. Each of us carries between three and eight genes which, if present in double dose in the offspring of two carriers of identical genes, would lead to severe genetic abnormality, or even to death, of the affected individual before or after birth. In view of the rapid medical advances in the treatment of such diseases, it is likely that affected individuals will be able to reproduce more frequently than in the past. Therefore, instead of a loss of genes due to death or sterility of the abnormal, the mutant gene will be transmitted to future generations in a slowly but steadily increasing frequency. This is leading the pessimists to predict that we will become a race of genetic cripples requiring a host of therapeutic crutches. The optimists, on the other hand, have great faith that the forces of natural evolution will continue to select favorably those individu-

From *Commonweal* 88 (May 17, 1968), pp. 257-61. Reprinted by permission of the author and publisher.

This paper was originally presented at a symposium sponsored by *Commonweal* and Marymount College, Tarrytown, New York.

als who are best adapted to the then current environment. It is important to remember in this context that the "natural" environment necessarily includes manmade medical, technical and social changes.

Since it appears that at least some of the aspects of evolution and a great deal of genetic planning will be in human and specifically in scientific hands, it is crucial at this relatively early stage to consider the ethical implications of these proposed maneuvers. Few scientists today doubt the feasibility of genetic engineering, and there is considerable danger that common use of this practice will be upon us before its ethical applications are defined.

A number of different methods have been proposed for the control and modification of human hereditary material. Some of these methods are meant to work on the population level, some on the family level and others directly on the affected individual. Interest in the alteration of the genetic pool of human populations originated shortly after the time of Mendel and Darwin in the latter part of the nineteenth century. The leaders were the English group of eugenicists headed by Galton. Eugenics is nothing more than planned breeding. This technique, of course, has been successfully used in the development of hybrid breeds of cattle, corn and other food products.

Human eugenics can be positive or negative. Positive eugenics is the preferential breeding of so-called superior individuals in order to improve the genetic stock of the human race. The most famous of the many proponents of positive eugenics was the late Nobel Prize-winner Herman J. Muller. He suggested that sperm banks be established from a relatively small number of donors, chosen by some appropriate panel, and that this frozen sperm remain in storage until some future panel had decided that the chosen donors truly represented desirable genetic studs. If the decision is favorable, a relatively large number of women would be inseminated with these samples of sperm; proponents of this method hope that a better world would result. The qualifications for such a donor would include high intellectual achievement and a socially desirable personality, qualities assumed to be affected by the genetic makeup of the individual, as well as an absence of obvious genetically determined physical anomalies.

A much more common effort is in the application of negative eugenics. This is defined as the discouragement or the legal prohibition of reproduction by individuals carrying genes leading to disease or disability. This can be achieved by genetic counseling or by sterilization, either on a voluntary or enforced basis. There are, however, quite divergent opinions as to which genetic traits are to be considered sufficiently disadvantageous to warrant the application of negative eugenics.

A diametrically opposite solution is that of euthenics, which is a modification of the environment in such a way as to allow the genetically abnormal individual to develop normally and to live a relatively normal life. Euthenics can be applied both medically and socially. The prescription of glasses for nearsighted individuals is an example of medical euthenics. Special schools for the deaf, a great proportion of whom are genetically abnormal, is an example of social euthenics. The humanitarianism of such efforts is obvious, but it is exactly these types of activities that have led to the concern of the pessimists who assume that evolution has elected for the best of possible variations in man and that further accumulations of genes considered abnormal can only lead to decline.

One of the most talked about advances for the future is the possibility of altering an individual's genetic complement. Since we are well on the way to understanding the genetic code, as well as to deciphering it, it is suggested that we can alter it. This code is written in a language of 64 letters, each being determined by a special arrangement of three out of four possible nucleotide bases. A chain of these bases is called deoxyribonucleic acid or DNA and makes up the genetic material of the chromosomes. If the altered letter responsible for an abnormal gene can be located and the appropriate nucleotide base substituted, the corrected message would again produce its normal product, which would be either a structurally or enzymologically functional protein.

Another method of providing a proper gene, or code word, to an individual having a defect has been suggested from an analysis of viral behavior in bacteria. It has long been known that certain types of viruses can carry genetic information from one bacterium to another or instruct a bacterium carrying it to produce what is essentially a viral product. Viruses are functional only when they live in a host cell. They use the host's genetic machinery to translate their own genetic codes. Viruses living parasitically in human cells can cause diseases such as poliomyelitis and have been implicated in the causation of tumors. Other viruses have been shown to live in cells and be reproduced along with the cells without causing damage either to the cell or to the organism. If such a harmless virus either produces a protein that will serve the function of one lacking in an affected individual, or if it can be made to carry the genetic material required for such functions into the cells of the affected individual, it could permanently cure the disease without additional therapy. If carried on to the next generation, it could even prevent the inheritance of the disease.

Transplanting Nuclei

An even more radical approach has been outlined by Lederberg. It has become possible to transplant whole nuclei, the structures which carry the DNA, from one cell to another. It has become easy to grow cells from various tissues of any individual in tissue culture. Such tissue cultures can be examined for a variety of genetic markers and thereby screened for evidence of new mutations. Lederberg suggests that it would be possible to use nuclei from such cells derived from known human individuals, again with favorable genetic traits, for the asexual human reproduction of replicas of the individuals whose nuclei are being used. For example, a nucleus from a cell of the chosen individual could be transplanted into a human egg whose own nucleus has been removed. This egg, implanted into a womb, could then divide just like a normal fertilized egg to produce an individual genetically identical to the one whose nucleus was used. One of the proposed advantages of such a method would be that, as in positive eugenics, one could choose the traits that appear to be favorable, and do so with greater efficiency by eliminating the somewhat randomly chosen female parent necessary for the sperm bank approach. Another advantage is that one can mimic what has developed in plants as a system for the preservation of genetic stability over limited periods of time. Many plants reproduce intermittently by such vegetative or parthenogenetic mechanisms, always followed by periods of sexual reproduction for the purpose of elimination of disadvantageous mutants and increase in variability.

Another possibility derives from two other technological advances. Tissue typing, similar to blood typing, and some immunological tricks have made it possible to transplant cells, tissues and organs from one individual to another with reasonably long-term success. Over the past few years scientists have also succeeded in producing cell hybrids containing some of the genetic material from each of two cell types either from two different species or two different individuals from the same species. Very recently Weiss and Green at New York University have succeeded in hybridizing normal human culture cells with cells from a long established mouse tissue culture line. Different products from such fusions contain varying numbers of human chromosomes and, therefore, varying amounts of human genes. If such hybrids can be produced which carry primarily that genetic information which is lacking or abnormal in an affected individual, transplantation of these cultured cells into the individual may produce a correction of his defect.

These are the proposed methods. It is now fair to consider the question of feasibility. Feasibility must be considered not only from a technical point of view; of equal importance are the effect of each of these methods on the evolution of the human population and the effect of evolution upon the efficacy of the method. In general, it can be stated that most of the proposed methods either are now or will in the not too distant future be technically possible. We are, therefore, not dealing with hypothesis in science fiction but with scientific reality. Let us consider each of the propositions independently.

Positive eugenics by means of artificial insemination from sperm banks has been practiced successfully in cattle for many years. Artificial insemination in man is an everyday occurrence. But what are some of its effects? There is now ample evidence in many species, including man, of the advantages for the population of individual genetic variation, mainly in terms of flexibility of adaptation to a changing environment. Changes in environment can produce drastic effects on some individuals, but a population which contains many genetic variations of that set of genes affected by the particular environmental change will contain numerous individuals who can adapt. There is also good evidence that individuals who carry two different forms of the same gene, that is, are heterozygous, appear to have an advantage. This is even true if that gene in double dose, that is, in the homozygous state, produces a severe disease. For example, individuals homozygous for the gene coding for sickle cell hemoglobin invariably develop sickle cell anemia which is generally fatal before the reproductive years. Heterozygotes for the gene are, however, protected more than normals from the effects of the most malignant form of malaria. It has been shown that women who carry the gene in single dose have a higher fertility in malarial areas than do normals. This effect is well known to agricultural geneticists and is referred to as hybrid vigor. Fertilization of many women by sperm from few men will have an adverse effect on both of these advantages of genetic variability since the population will tend to be more and more alike in their genetic characteristics. Also, selection for a few genetically advantageous factors will carry with it selection for a host of other genes present in the same individuals, genes whose effects are unknown when present in high numbers in the population. Therefore, the interaction between positive eugenics and evolution makes this method not feasible on its own.

Abnormal Offspring

Negative eugenics is, of course, currently practiced by most human geneticists. It is possible to detect carriers of many genes, which when inherited from both parents will produce abnormal offspring. Parents, both of whom carry such a gene, can be told that they have a one in four chance of producing such an abnormal child. Individuals who carry chromosomal translocations are informed that they have a high risk of producing offspring with congenital malformations and mental retardation. But how far can one carry out such a program? Some states have laws prescribing the sterilization of individuals who are mentally retarded to a certain degree. These laws are frequently based on false information regarding the heredity of the condition. The marriage of people with reduced intelligence is forbidden in some localities, again without adequate genetic information. While the effects of negative eugenics may be quite desirable in individual families with a high risk of known hereditary diseases, it is important to examine its effects on the general population.

These effects must be looked at individually for conditions determined by genes that express themselves in a single dose (dominant), in double dose (recessive) and those which are due to an interaction of many genes (polygenic inheritance). With a few exceptions, dominant diseases are rare and interfere severely with reproductive ability. They are generally maintained in the population by new mutations. Therefore, there is either no need or essentially no need for discouraging these individuals from reproduction. Any discouragement, if applicable, will be useful only within that family but will not have any significance for the general population. One possible exception is the severe neurological disorder, Huntington's chorea, which does not express itself until most of the patient's children are already born. In such a situation it may be useful to advise the child of an affected individual that he has a 50 percent chance of developing the disease and a 25 percent chance of any of his children being affected. Negative eugenics in such a case would at least keep the gene frequency at the level usually maintained by new mutations.

The story is quite different for recessive conditions. Although detection of the clinically normal carriers of these genes is currently possible only for a few diseases, the techniques are rapidly developing whereby many of these conditions can be diagnosed even if the gene is present only in single dose and will not cause the disease. Again, with any particular married couple it would be possible to advise them that they are both carriers of the gene and that any child of theirs would have a 25 percent chance of being affected. However, any attempt to decrease the gene frequency of these common genetic disorders in the population by prevention of fertility of all carriers would be doomed to failure. First, we all carry between three and eight of these genes in single doses. Secondly, for many of these conditions, the frequency in the population of carriers is about one in fifty or even greater. Prevention of fertility for even one of these disorders would stop a sizable proportion of the population from reproducing and for all of these disorders would prevent the entire human population from having any children. Reduction in fertility of a sizable proportion of the population would also prevent the passing on to future generations of a great number of favorable genes and would, therefore, interfere with the selective aspects of evolution which can only function to improve the population within a changing environment by selecting from a gene pool containing enormous variability. It has now been shown that in fact no two individuals, with the exception of identical twins, are likely to be genetically and biochemically identical, thereby allowing the greatest possible adaptation to changing environment and the most efficient selection of the fittest.

The most complex problem is that of negative eugenics for traits determined by polygenic inheritance. Characteristics inherited in this manner include many measurements that are distributed over a wide range throughout the population, such as height, birth weight and intelligence. The last of these can serve as a good example of the problems encountered. Severe mental retardation in a child is not infrequently associated with perfectly normal intelligence or in some cases even superior intelligence in the parents. These cases can, a priori, be assumed to be due to the homozygous state, in the child, of a gene leading to mental retardation, the parents representing heterozygous carriers. On the other hand, border-line mental retardation shows a high association with subnormal intelligence in other family members. This type of deficiency can be assumed to be due to polygenic factors, more of the pertinent genes in these families being of the variety that tends to lower intelligence. However, among the offspring of these families there is also a high proportion of individuals with normal intelligence and a sprinkling of individuals with superior intelligence.

All of these comments are made with the realization that our current measurements of intelligence are very crude and cannot be compared between different population groups. It is estimated that, on the whole, people with superior intelligence have fewer offspring than do those of average or somewhat below average intelligence. If people of normal intelligence were restricted to producing only two offspring and people of reduced intelligence were by negative eugenics prevented from having any offspring at all, the result, as has been calculated by the British geneticist, Lionel Penrose, would be a gradual shift downward in the mean intelligence level of the population. This is due to the lack of replacement of intellectually superior individuals from offspring of the majority of the population, that is, those not superior in intellect.

Current Possibilities

It can be seen, therefore, that neither positive nor negative eugenics can ever significantly improve the gene pool of the population and simultaneously allow for adequate evolutionary improvement of the human race. The only useful aspect of negative eugenics is in individual counseling of specific families in order to prevent some of the births of abnormal individuals. One recent advance in this sphere has important implications from both a genetic and a social point of view. It is now possible to diagnose genetic and chromosomal abnormalities in an unborn child by obtaining cells from the amniotic fluid in which the child lives in the mother. While the future may bring further advances, allowing one, then, to start treatment on the unborn child and to produce a functionally normal infant, the only currently possible solution is restricted to termination of particular pregnancies by therapeutic abortion. This is, of course, applied negative eugenics in its most extreme form.

Euthenics, the alteration of the environment to allow aberrant individuals to develop normally and to lead a normal life, is currently in use. Medical examples include special diets for children with a variety of inborn errors of metabolism who would, in the absence of such diets, either die or grow up mentally retarded. Such action, of course, requires very early diagnosis of these diseases, and programs are currently in effect to routinely examine newborns for such defects. Other examples include the treatment of diabetics with insulin and the provision of special devices for children with skeletal deformities. Social measures are of extreme importance in this regard. As has many times been pointed out by Dobzhansky, it is useless to plan for any type of genetic improvement if we do not provide an environment within which an individual can best use his strong qualities and obtain support for his weak qualities. One need only mention the availability of an environment conducive to artistic endeavor for Toulouse-Lautrec, who was deformed by an inherited disease.

The feasibility of alteration of an individual's genes by direct chemical change of his DNA is technically an enormously difficult task. Even if it became possible to do this, the chance of error would be enormous. Such an error, of course, would have the diametrically opposite effect of that desired; in other words, the individual would become even more abnormal. The introduction of corrective genetic material by viruses or transplantation of appropriately hybridized cells is technically predictable and, since it would be performed only in a single affected individual, would have no direct effect on the population. If it became widespread enough, it could, like euthenics, increase the frequency in the population of so-called abnormal genes, but if this treatment became a routine phenomenon, this would not develop into an evolutionarily disadvantageous situation. It must also be constantly kept in mind that medical advances are occurring at a much more rapid rate than any conceivable deterioration of the genetic endowment of man. It is, therefore, very likely that such corrective procedures will become commonplace long before there is a noticeable increase in the load of disadvantageous genes in the population.

The growing of human beings from cultured cells, while again possibly feasible, would on the other hand interfere with the action of evolutionary forces. There would be an increase, just as with positive eugenics, of a number of individuals who would be alike in their genetic complement with no opportunity for the high degree of genetic recombination which occurs during the formation of sperm and eggs and which is evident in the resultant progeny. This would diminish the adaptability of the population to changes in the environment and, of these genetic replicas were later permitted to return to sexual reproduction, would lead to a marked increase in homozygosity for a number of genes with the disadvantages pointed out before.

Who Will Be the Judges

We see, therefore, that many of the proposed techniques are feasible although not necessarily practical in producing their desired results. We may now ask the question of which of these are ethical from a humanistic point of view? Both positive and negative eugenics when applied to populations presume a judgment of what is genetically good and what is bad. Who will be the judges and where will the limit be between good and bad? We have had at least one example of a sad experience with eugenics in its application in Nazi Germany. This alone can serve as a lesson on the inability to separate science and politics. The most difficult decisions will come in defining the borderline cases. Will we breed against tallness because space requirements become more critical? Will we breed against nearsightedness because people with glasses may not make good astronauts? Will we forbid intellectually inferior individuals from procreating despite their proven ability to produce a number of superior individuals? Or should we rather provide an adequate environment for the offspring of such individuals to realize their full genetic potential?

C. C. Li, in his presidential address to the American Society of Human Genetics in 1960, pointed out the real fallacy in eugenic arguments. Man has continuously improved his environment to allow so-called inferior individuals to survive and reproduce. The movement into the cave and the putting on of clothes has protected the individual unable to survive the stress of the elements. Should we then consider that we have reached the peak of man's progress, largely determined by environmental improvements designed to increase fertility and longevity, and that any future improvements designed to permit anyone to live a normal life will only lead to deterioration? Nineteenth-century scientists, including such eminent biologists as Galton, firmly believed that this peak was reached in their time. This obviously fallacious reasoning must not allow a lapse in ethical considerations by the individual and by humanity as a whole, just to placate the genetic pessimists.

The tired axiom of democracy that all men are created equal must not be considered from the geneticist's point of view, since genetically all men are created unequal. Equality must be defined purely and simply as equality of opportunity to do what one is best equipped to do. When we achieve this, the forces of natural evolution will choose those individuals best adapted to this egalitarian environment. No matter how we change the genetic makeup of individuals, we cannot do away with natural selection. We must always remember that natural selection is determined by a combination of truly natural events and the artificial modifications which we are introducing into our environment in an exponentially increasing number.

With these points in mind, we can try to decide what in all of these methods is both feasible and ethical. I believe that the only logical conclusion is that all maneuvers of genetic engineering must be judged for each individual and, in each case, must take primary consideration of the rights of the individual. This is impossible by definition in any attempt at positive eugenics. Negative eugenics in the form of intelligent genetic counseling is the answer for some. Our currently unreasonable attitude about practicing negative eugenics by means of intelligent selection for therapeutic abortion must be changed. Basic to such a change is a more accurate definition of a living human being. Such restricted uses of negative eugenics will prevent individual tragedies. Correction of unprevented genetic disease, or that due to new mutation, by introduction of new genetic material may be one answer for the future; but until such a new world becomes universally feasible, we must on the whole restrict ourselves to environmental manipulations from both the points of view of allowing affected individuals to live normally and permitting each individual to realize his full genetic potential. There is no question that genetic engineering will come about. But both the scientists directly involved and, perhaps more important, the political and social leaders of our civilization must exercise utmost caution in order to prevent genetic, evolutionary and social tragedies.

Part II

Abortion on Demand

Widespread public argument over whether mankind should shape its own genetic structure may lie in the future. Other life-and-death issues have already penetrated the public mind: "Abortion is murder," "It's *my* body," "A fetus is not a person." The arguments rage over abortion with intense passion, and the Supreme Court decision of January 1973 declaring all state laws that forbid abortion null and void only added to the polarization of the struggle. Election campaigns are won and lost on the issue; state referendums appear on ballots; legal battles involving doctors are argued by untiring lawyers, and two constitutional amendments are being shaped.

In the following selections the less emotional arguments are presented, although we have tried to offer various aspects of the issue as fairly and objectively as possibly. Mildred B. Beck argues the case of the unwanted child: it is better to terminate a pregnancy than to bring a child into a world of neglect, abandonment, or injury. Following this plea, Betty Sarvis and Hyman Rodman present a detailed analysis of the attitudes of different groups toward abortion—and point out that no group lacks the motivation to practice birth control but many lack the information. John T. Noonan, Jr. cautions against using personal abstractions when looking at a legal or moral issue, and tries to avoid old, worn-out arguments while setting forth his point of view. Nick Thimmesch reassures us that we are not headed toward a Nazi society thanks to the checks presented by the press, legislators, doctors, lawyers, and the clergy. John A. Miles also looks at the larger issue. Miles writes that the real matter under discussion is not just abortion, but the national response to the coming technology of social science. We end with an account of a legal case in Boston. Richard Landau points out that a corporation is considered a "person" with rights to equal protection according to the Fourteenth Amendment; therefore, should not a fetus have the same protection?

8

The Destiny
of the Unwanted Child

Mildred B. Beck

Much has been written about the consequences of unwanted pregnancy for the pregnant woman, the father, and others significantly related to them. Strikingly little, by contrast, has been written—or is known—about the fate of the child compelled to be born against the wishes of his mother, his father, or both. Yet he is, to say the least, an interested party. Ironically, though he has many spokesmen, they do not speak with one voice. Nor do these spokesmen truly represent him, for they are self-designated, express their personal views, and fight for what *they* believe is good for children. When the "good" is described in diametrically conflicting terms, however, it is desirable wherever possible to separate fact from fancy, conjecture from evidence, and wishful thinking from reality.

I address myself here to what is known to be true, even within the limited state of present knowledge, and I will suggest areas of needed research. As a necessary preliminary, I define "compulsory pregnancy"* to mean a particular pregnancy, incurred by chance or by plan, which for any reason whatsoever is steadfastly and unequivocally unwanted by the pregnant woman, but which she is compelled by external circumstances to carry to term. The qualifying words are intended to preclude the transitory ambivalence that may have assailed virtually every pregnant woman since the beginning of time.

Originally published as "The Destiny of the Unwanted Child: The Issue of Compulsory Pregnancy," in *Abortion and the Unwanted Child*, ed. Carl Reiterman, pp. 59-71. Copyright © 1971 by Springer Publishing Co. Reprinted by permission.

*I am indebted for this term to Garrett Hardin who, to the best of my knowledge, coined it. Its currency is a mark of its usefulness.

There are extremely important differences between women who say "I *never* want to become pregnant" and those who say "I do not want *this* pregnancy" for one or more of the following reasons:

1. I am told that my child, on the basis of medical findings, stands a substantial chance of being severely deformed or retarded. (This includes rubella victims, cases where the fetus is at risk for genetic reasons, cases where the parent has used damaging drugs, etc.).

2. The doctor warned me against another pregnancy because I have a severe heart condition (or some other life-threatening or life-shortening disability).

3. I can barely care for the three (four, five, six. . .) children I already have.

4. My husband has just returned from Vietnam and he is under an incredible strain that I don't understand. I just can't look after our other kids and him, too. . . and, my God, another baby!

5. This baby is cursed, just as all my father's other children are.[1]

6. We've practiced birth control effectively until now and our children are spaced just as we wanted them. I don't want this baby; in fact, I just can't raise another.

7. You aren't going to let her have this kid, are you? She's only twelve herself!

8. I never really wanted a baby; I just wanted to see if I could get pregnant. I hate kids!

9. We'll *have* to marry if I am forced to have this baby because my parents insist. But they can have the baby and you can have the father. I won't live with him for a minute!

Highly responsible persons who seek to terminate a pregnancy do so because of concern for the outcome for themselves, the child-to-be, and others close to them whose lives are adversely affected by the unwanted pregnancy. There also are women, characterized by varying degrees of "immaturity." Assuming that society has an interest in reducing uncontrolled, and some forms of uncontrollable, sexual behavior, how can this be done? By compelling a woman to carry to term an unwanted pregnancy, placing in her custody an absolutely helpless and hapless infant? Is there any evidence to suggest that this is a successful method? And what is the cost to the infant? Erik Erikson, in *Childhood and*

Society, contends that "the firm establishment of enduring patterns. . . of basic trust. . . is the first task of the ego, and thus the first task for maternal care. But. . . the amount of trust derived from earliest infantile experience [depends] on *the quality of the maternal relationship.* Mothers create a sense of trust in their children. . . . This forms the basis in the child for a sense of identity which will later combine a sense of being 'all right,' or being oneself, and of becoming what other people trust one will become."[2] One must, then, inquire *whose* interests are served by compulsory pregnancy, and into the outcome for each of the principals.

In this presentation, the "unwanted child" is seen as the product of a compulsory (unwanted) pregnancy, whether or not the mother seeks a legal or an illegal abortion, or whether or not she attempts to abort herself. Legal abortions still are for the few who have luck, influential friends, money, or who can borrow substantial sums. Available statistics indicate that each year some 10,000 women have legal abortions; estimates of the incidence of illegal and self-induced abortion range between 200,000 and 1,200,000. In addition, an unknown number of women make unsuccessful attempts at inducing abortion, and in these cases one can only speculate about the damage they may have done to themselves or to the child.

The unwanted child is characterized by one or more of the following:

1. He has biological parents only. Although he is rarely, often never seen by his parents after birth, he is not necessarily released for adoption or other long-term care. At times the parent cannot be found, or refuses to become involved in any way in the care of, or planning for, the child or, even when the law permits the legal termination of parenthood, withholds consent. (Agencies sometimes fail to terminate parental rights, even when it is legally permissible, because an adoptive home cannot be found, perhaps because of race, religion, or because the child is physically or mentally handicapped.)

2. He is abandoned: wrapped in a paper bag or newspaper, and left in a refuse can; or perhaps left, unfed, and sometimes injured, on a doorstep, or in a hallway, or with a "sitter," often a person relatively unknown to the parents.

3. He is neglected or abused in the sense that, if the child were

brought to the attention of the courts, there would ensue a legal finding of neglect or abuse. Here we include children suffering from severe malnutrition although the mother does not lack knowledge of nutrition, and there is no evidence of financial need; the infant or young child who is left for days on end with some vague provision for someone to look in on him from time to time; the children left for prolonged periods in so-called well-baby wards of hospitals, or in shelters, or in emergency foster care when there is no demonstrable evidence of need or when the mother offers one excuse after another for failing to provide for the child in any way whatsoever.

Such are the circumstances of the lives of unwanted children. A few details complete this unhappy picture. Many of the mothers of these children have tried to get contraceptive help, and later an abortion, but to no avail. Many of these women are mentally and emotionally ill or retarded. Some are drug addicts or alcoholics. With shocking frequency, they were, more often than not, themselves the object of childhood abuse. Another group, of unknown size, present a curious phenomenon. Dr. Gerald Caplan of the Harvard School of Public Health found that young children were brought to a child guidance clinic by mothers who—except in their relationship to the patient—were warm, generous, good mothers. During the course of treatment almost every mother "confessed" that she tried to abort the patient, and—considering the nature of these efforts—she was sure the child was damaged. She responds to the child as though it had actually been impaired by her; furthermore, she comes to believe that the child knows what she "tried to do to him," and she then ascribes to the child a deliberate talent for meanness and revenge in his response to her. What a tragic penalty must be paid by the unwitting victim! Clearly, where unwanted children are concerned, we must ask not only who punishes whom, but also how much society itself is *compelled* to pay for the human suffering that it unintentionally imposes.

Lacking definitive studies of the outcome, over periods of time, of compulsory pregnancies, contending factions are in a position to defend cherished theories. It is possible, for example, that a child born of a compulsory pregnancy may become the most loved and treasured of children. And a few of these children may indeed become Beethovens or Michelangelos. But how many of these potential geniuses disappear into anaclitic depressions after spending months in institutional well-baby wards? And how many lesser lights are dimmed or extinguished by neglect? In fact, many thousands of babies and young children become unplaceable *after* society has intervened in their behalf because suitable foster and adoptive homes are not available to them until months or years after they are first needed.

Historical Perspective

A few statistics may be illuminating. According to Dr. Robert Hall, abortion before "quickening" was not proscribed by religious groups in the Western world until 1803. The first anti-abortion law in the United States was not passed until 1835. And it was not until 1869 that, for the first time, early abortion was viewed as murder by the Catholic Church.

Until 1966, forty-five American states defined abortion as unlawful unless it was necessary to preserve the *life* and, in five states and the District of Columbia, the *health* of the mother. Interestingly, the abortion rate was the same in all states, despite the more liberal interpretation in the latter five states, probably because competent and concerned physicians everywhere have often elected to protect the *health* of the woman irrespective of the law. But concern for the welfare of the infant, despite such known hazards as rubella and certain genetic disorders, was not an indication for abortion in any state. Yet long before 1966 physicians aborted women for these and other reasons in keeping with the dictates of their professional and ethical beliefs and their deep concern for human welfare. Still, in most states today, conscientious and law-abiding physicians must continue to make the terrible choice between permitting virtually inevitable tragedy or of skirting the law and practicing medicine that is in accord with modern medical knowledge.

We should remember that public relations and promotional techniques were not invented by Madison Avenue. Our predecessors had some effective techniques of their own. They elicited— only too successfully—the offices of the church and related institutions, reinforcing all with the power of the law. The problem today is: How do we reform or repeal laws that have fulfilled their mission, and proceed to take account of new knowledge, accumulated experience, and contemporary values?

At the moment we often find ourselves in untenable positions. For instance, it is extremely difficult to demonstrate that a woman is at risk, physically or mentally, as some of the liberalized abortion laws demand. Certifying that a pregnant woman's life or health is at risk "temporarily or with medical certainty" as a direct consequence of the pregnancy asks physicians and psychiatrists to be clairvoyant. Yet, the danger to the physical and mental well-being of the mother and child is far greater, certainly over time, than the law recognizes. Worst of all, the laws are applied capriciously, inequitably and—not infrequently—hypocritically. Here attention is called to the testimony of those who serve on, or are associated with, hospital abortion committees. As for the discriminatory application of the law, Robert Hall has reported that "private patients get hospital abortions four times as often as ward patients."[3]

Unwanted children have been born throughout recorded history, but they have been dealt with differently from one period to another. It should be remembered that the Society for the Prevention of Cruelty to *Animals* first appeared in England in 1824, and in the United States in 1866. The Society for the Prevention of Cruelty to *Children* was established in the United States five years later. This is only one of countless indications throughout recorded history illustrating, not that we care more about animals than children, but that most human beings cannot bring themselves to reflect upon the depth and the extent of the suffering of children.

In the past unwanted children were dealt with much more forthrightly though not always more inhumanely than today. Infanticide, *by contrast* not the worst fate that can befall an infant, is described from earliest times. As recently as the eighteenth and nineteenth centuries, overt as well as disguised infanticide was commonplace. William Langer, discussing conditions in Europe, makes this plain:

> In the cities it was common practice to confide babies to old woman nurses or caretakers. The least offense of the "Angelmakers," as they were called. . . , was to give children gin to keep them quiet. [According to Disraeli], "Laudanum and treacle, administered in the shape of some popular elixir, affords these innocents a brief taste of the sweets of existence and, keeping them quiet, prepares them for the silence of their impending grave. . . . Infanticide is practiced as extensively and as legally in England as it is on the banks of the Ganges. . . .

The middle and late 18th Century was marked by a startling rise in the rate of illegitimacy [and] so many of the unwanted babies were being abandoned, smothered or otherwise disposed of that Napoleon in 1811 decreed that foundling hospitals should be provided with a turntable device, so that babies could be left at these institutions without the parent being recognized or subjected to embarrassing questions. This convenient arrangement was imitated in many countries and was taken full advantage of. . . . Of the thousands of children thus abandoned, more than half were the offspring of married couples. . . .

Most of the children died within a short time, either of malnutrition or neglect. . . . In some of the Italian hospitals the mortality ran to 80 or 90 percent. In Paris the Maison de la Couche reported that of 4,779 babies admitted in 1818, 2,370 died in the first three months and another 956 within the first year. . . . Many contemporaries denounced [this system] as legalized infanticide, and one. . . suggested that the foundling hospitals post a sign reading, "Children killed at Government expense."

In light of the available data one is almost forced to admit that the proposal, seriously advanced at the time, that unwanted babies be painlessly asphyxiated in small gas chambers was definitely humanitarian.[4]

How do unwanted children fare today? Are we asking the right questions, the basic questions as to *why* we have so many? Have we investigated the fate of these children from the moment the *unwanting mother* perceives that she is pregnant? And what responsibility do those who staunchly fight for the rights of the fetus assume, *postnatally,* to ensure the fulfillment of these rights? Finally, since society dictates most of the conditions under which we live, what does society do for the unwanted child?

We may never get accurate figures on the number of unplanned and unwanted pregnancies and children in the United States, but we have clues. According to Dr. Alan Guttmacher, President of Planned Parenthood/World Population, four out of five American couples practice some form of birth control after a first child is born but, because of contraceptive failure due to unreliability of the method or careless use, about half of their subsequent pregnancies are unplanned.[5] And in 1967, 318,000, or slightly more than 9 percent of all United States births were illegitimate, and approximately 40 percent of these births were to mothers

15-19 years of age.[6] In all probability the recorded number of illegitimate births would be substantially increased were it not for false birth certificates. Add babies born to couples whose marriages were enforced by parental or other pressures, and the presumed number of unwanted infants rises sharply.[7]

If it were true, as some assert, that the unwanted infant usually becomes wanted after birth, why are so many babies and young children abandoned? Why are more than 300,000 American children, according to Child Welfare League and U.S. Children's Bureau estimates, in foster care on any given day? How does it happen that 100,000 of these children are trapped in foster care and have virtually no hope of returning to their own homes—if ever there was one? And how can we explain the 46 percent of the children currently in foster care who are there because of "parental neglect, abuse, or exploitation?" As for the others, broken homes, economic problems, disabling physical and mental disabilities of one or both parents characterize nearly all as "orphans of the living."

If prenatal care is of value in ensuring a healthy mother and infant, its absence is a loss. But how many women, bent on getting an abortion, are likely to seek prenatal care or to avail themselves of it even when it is offered? We have evidence that an unwanted pregnancy sets a destructive process in motion. One need only talk with unwillingly pregnant women—married or unmarried, too young to be a "teenager" or old enough to be menopausal, rich or poor, of any skin hue. Hear them describe what they have tried in order to induce abortion; what they will yet do if worse comes to worst; and note their despair, rage, and their sense of utter defeat. The methods that have been employed by desperate women are documented in Norman Hime's classic *Medical History of Contraception*.[8] We merely report here that some of these methods are almost beyond the reader's capacity to bear.

Many women, despite incredibly savage and damaging efforts to induce an abortion, fail and come to term. If, as some contend, it is the pregnant woman and not the fetus that suffers prenatal deprivations of all kinds, what kind of mother—physically and psychologically—will she be to that completely dependent and helpless infant? Conversely, if the fetus is susceptible to damage and shock, what degree of permanent harm will have been done to him? As long as we continue to deny abortions to women who want them, we have an obligation to ascertain the fetus's chance of successful survival of the pregnancy as well as the days and months that follow. The defenders of the premise that a child has a right to a decent life of dignity and fulfillment are, in my judgment, obligated to ensure that these conditions are met. Otherwise, the fetus's defenders may condemn him, postnatally, to neglect, abuse, lifelong institutionalization, or the threat of infanticide.

We have long deplored the paucity of data on the outcome of unwanted pregnancy. The allegation that it is impossible to study the outcome of unwanted pregnancies and denied abortions is subject to serious challenge.

If one recalls Victor Hugo's observation that "nothing is as powerful as an idea whose time has come," one will not be surprised that recently a substantial number of articles, studies and unpublished manuscripts have been addressed to the fate of the unwanted child.[9] Some of these documents first appeared in obscure scientific or small-audience journals because of the controversial nature of the subject.

On the matter of studying the outcome of denied abortions, the opportunities now only wait to be grasped. As an example, in Maryland there are far more legitimate requests for abortion than current resources can handle, and the growing number of pleas for these services from outside the state must, of necessity, be denied. Why not follow up these women in their home states to ascertain what happens where abortion has been denied? Why not look into the outcome for the hundreds of school-age youngsters who remain in school but who are compelled to come to term with unwanted pregnancies? Further, why not attempt to ascertain what has happened to a woman, known to be pregnant, who suddenly no longer is? Can all these noncompleted pregnancies be subsumed under the rubric of spontaneous abortion? Or did all these women go out of town, deliver their babies in secret, and leave them for an unknown person or agency to care for? What is in store for the babies whose unwanted lives we succeed in saving? Oughtn't we to know? Can we justify not knowing? The staggering cost in money, in alarmingly depleted resources for good foster and adoptive homes and for acceptable group care programs is a stiff penalty not only for the woman who has been forced to bear a child against her will or best judgment, but also for the child. Another highly important researchable area pertains to child abuse, a problem of international concern. All fifty American states have passed laws providing for mandatory reporting of presumed instances of child abuse, and the reporting agents—usually physicians, hospitals, and child care institutions—are assured protection against libel suits. The fact that these laws are not producing the hoped-for results suggests the need for prompt study and appropriate action. We should remember that since the majority of abusive parents have been the victims of abuse in their own youth, it follows that victimized children in their turn may become victimizing adults.

According to Drs. Helfer and Kempe, in the United States in 1967 "tens of thousands of children were severely battered or killed." Dr. David Gil, of Brandeis University, notes that reported rates of child abuse represent "an unknown fraction of actual incidence rates."[10] This under-reporting, according to Katherine B. Oettinger, is due in part to the fact that "there are few topics in modern life that are more repugnant. . . than the abuse of a child by the very persons entrusted with his care. Yet the fact is that some people of every socioeconomic, educational, religious, and geographical background in our society continue to abuse their children." Further, even in states like New York, where legislation provides for mandatory reporting of suspected cases of child abuse, under-reporting is said to be due to the alarming contention that "hospitals and doctors have begun to say there is nothing to be gained by reporting these tragedies. Society doesn't seem ready to do anything about them anyway."[11]

The Battered Child is not an easy book to read. But to cite a few more findings, Drs. Steele and Pollack studied sixty families intensively where significant abuse of infants and small children under the age of three had occurred.[12] (Murder is not included in this sample because the authors hold that "direct murder of children is an entirely different phenomenon and is instigated during a single, impulsive act by people who are clearly psychotic.") The parents included:

> laborers, farmers, blue-collar workers, white-collar workers and top professional people. Some were in poverty, some were relatively wealthy, but most were in-between. . . . Educational achievement ranged from partial grade school to advanced postgraduate degrees. . . . Intellectual ability ranged from IQs in the 70's to superior ratings of 130. . . . The parents ranged from 18 to 40 years of age, the great majority being in the twenties. . . . The great majority were in

relatively stable marriages. . . . Religious affiliations included
Catholic, Jewish and Protestant. . . . Most families were
Anglo-Saxon Americans. . . . True alcoholism was not a
problem except in one family and many were total abstain-
ers. . . . The actual attack on the infant is usually made by
one parent. . . . The mother was the attacker in fifty
instances, the father in seven, in one family both parents
attacked and in two instances, it was difficult to determine
which parent was primarily involved.

The parents, on psychiatric examination, were found to be
suffering from "hysteria, hysterical psychosis, obsessive-compul-
sive neurosis, anxiety states, depression, schizoid personality traits,
schizophrenia, character neurosis and so on" (p. 108).

There are, of course, many complex factors that contribute to
child abuse. But few investigators make a systematic attempt to
discover how many of the abusive parents had given clues that the
pregnancy was unwanted. In fact, many parents feared the
pregnancy because they sensed their uncontrollable aggression
toward the coming child. For example, "a pre-maritally conceived
pregnancy or one which comes too soon after the birth of a
previous child. . . may be perceived as public reminders of sexual
transgression or as extra, unwanted burdens" (p. 129).

Radbill, in "A History of Child Abuse and Infanticide" (p. 3)
traces the maltreatment of children from earliest times. Infanticide
has been practiced for population control, the control of family
size, because the child was illegitimate, for economic reasons,
because of the mother's "illness, death, youth, debauchery, or
demands made upon her by the needs of older siblings, . . . or
because of the taboo which kept the mother away from the
embraces of her husband during the lactation period, or [the
superstitious fear] that twins, monstrous births or congenital
defects frequently bode evil. . . . During the period of the Caesars,
infanticide, always legal in Rome, received the approbation of
philosophers like Seneca."[13]

Abuse of children is tragic. But it could be reduced by
eliminating compulsory pregnancy, and by helping people to
conceive, bear, and cherish children who are wanted and welcomed.

In conclusion I would like to cite a viewpoint of special
importance in a democracy, as expressed by R. E. L. Masters:

Those of us who claim to be reasonable men and women, who are dedicated to bringing about a maximum application of reason to the regulation of human conduct, must not hesitate when it is necessary to collide with the defenders of prohibitions, even in those areas where they are passionate and fanatical to a dangerous and sometimes pathological degree.

In the nuclear age it is more essential than ever that superstition and ignorance be overcome. The blind emotivity of fanaticism has become too menacing to be tolerable. The irrational, where discernible in moral codes and political systems, must be firmly weeded out. The time for taboo has passed. In the modern world, freedom is to be tampered with only when society's requirements are both reasonable and compelling; and then to the slightest degree possible. The soundest and most urgent of motives must underlie any attempt to tell men and women how to behave and how not to behave. When the forces of totalitarianism are so powerful, the correct choice is to attempt to *expand* the areas of liberty.

The compelling reasons advanced for prohibitions must have contemporary, not antique, validity. Appeals to various of humanity's gods, prophets, and religions will not do. Having rejected magic and superstition generally, we may scarcely with intelligence and integrity continue to cling to prohibitions transparently magical and superstitious in origin, unless those prohibitions may now be otherwise and adequately justified. For those who wish to base their conduct upon the revelations and edicts of this god or that one, there is the ever-available concept of sin; but only in a theocracy should what is sinful be also necessarily criminal.[14]

Notes

1. In *Child Victims of Incest,* the American Humane Association has estimated an incidence of 832,000 cases of incest in the United States in a fifteen-year period.

2. New York: W. W. Norton, 2nd edition. rev. 1963, p. 249. Emphasis added.

3. *Saturday Review,* December 7, 1968, p. 79.

4. "Disguised Infanticide," *American Historical Review* 69 (1963).

5. "The Tragedy of the Unwanted Child," *Parents' Magazine,* June 1964.

6. U. S. Department of Health, Education, and Welfare, *Trends in Illegitimacy: United States 1940-1965* (February 1968), p. 5.

7. Please note that Dr. Charles F. Westoff in an address to the annual meeting of Planned Parenthood—World Population on October 28, 1969, "Extent of Unwanted Fertility in the United States," estimated the number of unwanted children born in the United States to be 800,000 per annum.

8. New York: Gamut Press, 1963.

9. H. Forssman and I. Thuwe, "En Socialpsykiatrisk efterundersökning av 120 barn födda efter auslag på abortframställning" (Mental Health and Social Adjustment of 120 Children Born After Application for Therapeutic Abortion Refused), *Nord. psykiat.* 14 (1960), pp. 265-79.

10. "Incidence of Child Abuse and Demographic Characteristics of Persons Involved," chapter 2 in Helfer and Kempe, eds., *The Battered Child* (Chicago: University of Chicago Press, 1968).

11. Private communication to the writer from a distinguished New York philanthropist, long associated with the child care field.

12. "A Psychiatric Study of Parents Who Abused Infants and Small Children," in Helfer and Kempe, eds., *The Battered Child*, p. 103.

13. Helfer and Kempe. *The Battered Child*, p. 3.

14. R. E. L. Masters, *Patterns of Incest* (The Julian Press, 1963).

9

Social and Cultural Aspects of Abortion: Class and Race

Betty Sarvis and Hyman Rodman

The knowledge that individuals have about abortion and their attitudes and behavior are greatly influenced by the social and cultural context. If one wants to predict the circumstances under which a person regards abortion as moral or immoral, or whether a woman experiences relief or guilt after an abortion, the most important item of information would be the sociocultural interpretation of abortion. Social class, race, religion, place of residence, and marital status are among the social variables that influence a person's access to, use of, and attitudes toward abortion services and alternatives to abortion. The rapid changes that have taken place in the United States in the past decade also underline time as an important variable.

Sexual Behavior, Contraception, and Pregnancy

Abortion presumably terminates an unwanted pregnancy, but as Pohlman and Pohlman (1969:181–95) point out, defining "unwanted" and "wanted" can be a complex undertaking. Some people, for example, proceed as though pregnancy out of wedlock is usually unwanted (Meier, 1961:144–46) while others assume that it is usually wanted (Harrison, 1969:366–67). An "unwanted" pregnancy can be transformed into one that is "wanted": if the pregnancy is unwanted only because the woman is unmarried, she may marry; or the woman may adapt herself to the idea of continuing an unwanted pregnancy, eventually coming to want it. Because of changed circumstances, a wanted pregnancy can also become unwanted. An unwanted pregnancy may be carried to

From *The Abortion Controversy* (New York: Columbia University Press, 1974), 2d ed., pp. 153-64. Reprinted by permission of the authors and publisher.

term, at which point the mother may keep the child or give the child up for adoption or foster care. Although it is often difficult to know what is meant by an unwanted or wanted pregnancy or whether an unwanted pregnancy has really become wanted, clearly there are several alternate ways of responding to an unwanted pregnancy. Within the United States the influence of social class and racial background upon various responses to an unwanted pregnancy has aroused a good deal of controversy.*

Many national and regional studies carried out in the last twenty years indicate that the poor, blacks, and the less educated want about the same number of children as others in society. Blacks, in fact, want as few or even fewer children than whites. Despite the desire for relatively small families within these groups, the studies also established that they wind up having larger families than they desire. The largest excess in fertility is to be found among the poor, nonwhites, and the less educated. Why do these groups have a greater proportion of excess fertility (children beyond the desired number)? In the first place, comparing blacks to whites, black women on the average engage in sexual relations earlier than white women and have their first child at a younger age than white women. The earlier birth of the first child for the black woman can have an important bearing upon her educational or occupational plans, and several investigators have suggested the limitations of using maternity wards as the major locations for providing contraceptive information. As Campbell (1968:238) has said, "it may be more important to delay the first child than to prevent the seventh." The responsibilities of caring for the first child, whether in or out of marriage, can effectively interfere with work and school plans and thus depress a woman's life chances. Beyond the early premarital years, little difference is found in the frequency of sexual intercourse, with whites possibly having a somewhat higher average frequency than blacks. For all married couples in the 1965 National Fertility Study, Westoff and Westoff (1971) report an average monthly frequency of sexual intercourse

*See the following references for information on racial and social class differences with respect to sexual behavior, contraception, and pregnancy: Gebhard et al. (1958); Freedman et al. (1959); Rainwater (1960, 1965, 1970); Hill and Jaffe (1967); Whelpton et al. (1966); Bogue (1967, 1970, 1970a); Schulz (1969); Baird (1970); Cartwright (1970); Zelnik and Kantner (1970); Ladner (1971); Presser (1971); Ryan (1971); Ryder and Westoff (1971); Westoff and Westoff (1971); and Staples (1972).

of 6.8 for whites and 6.3 for blacks.

Another important finding of the fertility studies suggests that the excess fertility among the poor, nonwhites, and the less educated stems from their less frequent and less effective use of contraceptives. Ryder and Westoff (1971:349–54), for example, report that although at each birth order a higher percentage of blacks do not want additional children, a lower percentage are actually using contraceptives. They also report much higher percentages of failure among blacks who use contraceptives than whites. Although they found little difference by educational level on the desire for children, those who did not complete high school show much lower percentages using contraceptives, and among those using them a consistently higher rate of failure. Some studies do not go beyond pointing out the different patterns of contraceptive use and effectiveness, but other have tried to explain the differences. The most convincing explanations have pointed out that the higher fertility groups have less knowledge of and less access to contraceptives, especially to the most effective methods (pills, IUDs). Once women make contact with a family planning clinic they tend to become effective contraceptive users. Several studies dealing with the experience of low-income women who have received contraceptives at clinics report very high percentages of women who use them successfully. Phyllis Champion's (1967:126) study led her to take an optimistic view of the potential for successful contraceptive use by low-income black couples. Her sample of low-income black women "showed no less perseverence, no 'weaker motivation' or no more evidence of 'improvidence' than Planned Parenthood has encountered elsewhere with its white patients from middle-class and suburban areas." Another recent study by Feldman et al. (1971) is also optimistic about the continued and successful use of contraceptives by low-income women. In this study, as in the Champion study, the women had voluntarily attended Planned Parenthood clinics and were taking the contraceptive pill.

To what extent would the equal and easy availability of the pill (or other effective contraceptives) to all racial and income groups reduce the racial and social class discrepancies in unwanted pregnancies for the population at large? It is only since 1967, when the federal government included family planning in its anti-poverty program, that there has been any substantial movement toward providing the poor with equal access to family planning services. Jaffe (1972) has suggested that these family planning services have contributed toward the substantial decline in fertility that has been observed in recent years among the poor. Jaffe warns that much still needs to be done since a large demand for family planning services exists not only among the poor, but also among the near-poor who cannot afford private medical care yet who do not qualify for subsidized care. The extension of family planning services to all who want them but who now find them inaccessible is likely to further decrease the higher fertility rate of the poor. No group lacks motivation to practice birth control. As Dorothy Millstone (1972:23) so vividly expressed it: "The coalition Mrs. Sanger was fighting for now exists. The fact is everyone wants protection against unwanted childbirth: the AFDC mother, the middle- and upper-class matron, the corporate executive, the high school cheerleader, the college man and woman, the hippie—everybody. They don't have to be bribed or coerced to accept it."

Obviously, less use of contraceptives and higher rates of contraceptive failure result in larger percentages of unwanted pregnancies. A woman can carry the child to term, keep the child or place the child for adoption or foster care, or she can abort. Public concern has focused on the unmarried woman who keeps her child—that is, the infamous illegitimate births—and especially upon the higher proportion of illegitimate births among the poor and blacks than among the middle class and whites. As several investigators have pointed out, far more white women than black women opt for a "shotgun" marriage which converts an illegitimate pregnancy into a legitimate birth (Gebhard et al., 1958; Coombs et al., 1970; Rains, 1971; Ryan, 1971). With respect to adoption, Rains (1971) observes that illegitimately pregnant white women are more likely to receive help. More cynically Ryan (1971:102) assesses the adoption prospects for black and white babies: "Black babies and babies of mixed racial parentage, who are classified as black, are a less readily marketed product in the adoption exchange; they are lumped together with those having genuine defects. In the adoption market, the best-seller is the infant who is fair, structurally intact, and mechanically sound."

At all points of choice the middle-class white woman usually has more alternatives than the lower-class black woman. The white woman has greater access to contraception, abortion, forced marriage, and adoption. Some evidence suggests that blacks prefer illegitimate childbirth to abortion (Rodman et al., 1969:319), but this evidence has too often been extended to mean that lower-class and black women "are accepting and philosophical about bearing out-of-wedlock babies because welfare provides such a simple and practical economic solution to the problem. Thus, there is supposed to be a direct relation between the prevalence of bastards and the expanding rolls of Aid to Families with Dependent Children" (Ryan, 1971:92). In the first place Ryan (1971:103, 106) finds that "only a minority of unmarried mothers depend on public assistance," and "to suggest that anyone—or at least more than a tiny handful of erratic or disturbed persons—would choose the bitter existence of AFDC as a way of life except as a last resort, is to demonstrate ignorance either of the basic nature of humanity, or of what life is like on AFDC." The lower-class woman has fewer alternatives to an unwanted pregnancy and has therefore "stretched" her values in order to grant greater acceptability to the behavior patterns, such as illegitimacy, to which she is often led by force of circumstances (Rodman, 1963). In contrast, the middle-class woman is able to maintain a highly negative attitude toward illegitimacy because she can rely almost completely upon abortion, adoption, or a forced marriage to conceal premarital pregnancies.

Changes in adoption practices, in access to services, and in attitudes are going to alter this situation. The adoption picture is changing: adoption agencies urge people to adopt older children, previously excluded groups (singles and older couples) adopt, more women have abortions, and more unmarried white women than previously keep their illegitimate children. This all adds up to fewer children to be adopted by more people, and some observers have expressed concern over a "shortage" of children to adopt. For a long time the unwed mother and her child have been singled out as major "social problems" while other possible targets in the arena—unequal access to resources or services, arbitrary restrictions of adoption agencies, or forced marriages and their associated marital difficulties—have for the most part escaped public rebuke. As Prudence Rains (1971:175-76) says,

> The definition of illegitimacy as a social problem, a social problem with sources usually traced to sexual behavior, is something of a political act. For it is a definition which not only tends to deflect attention from social inequalities in access to other solutions to the problem of pregnancy—

primarily abortion—but also supplies support for the questionable view that having and keeping an illegitimate child is the least acceptable solution to the problem of pregnancy.

If abortion becomes available to all women, it can be a widely used alternative to illegitimacy. But Rains (1971:177) also expresses the view of many when she says that "it is difficult to sustain the position that abortion is ethically or socially preferable to illegitimacy as a solution to the problem of illegitimate pregnancy." In the end she pleads for social policies "which will address the problems of unwed mothers" (Rains, 1971:178). It is, however, politically dangerous to endorse expanded services to unwed mothers and U.S. welfare legislation addressed to them is typically punitive.

Race, Class, and Abortion

If we use excess fertility as a criterion, then the poor, blacks, and other minority groups are the largest potential users of abortion. Two major lines of evidence in the literature during the 1950s and 1960s reveal that these groups do not have equal access to abortion facilities. First, higher rates of abortions were reported for private patients than for public or general service patients. Second is the higher rate of abortions reported for white patients than for nonwhites or other minority groups. Table 1 summarizes a selection of this evidence from four different studies based on the years 1951 to 1970.

It is clear from Table 1 that the rate of legal abortions per 1,000 live births is considerably higher for whites than for nonwhites (principally blacks). These differences are consistent throughout, for New York City, for the state of Georgia, and for the United States samples. The rate of legal abortions for Puerto Ricans in New York City, during the same time period, is even lower than the rate for blacks (Gold et al., 1965:966). With respect to the abortion rates for voluntary hospitals in New York City, Table 1 shows that the rate for private service patients is consistently higher than the rate for general service patients. The difference is even more pronounced, for each of the reported time periods, if we compare the abortion rate at private hospitals with the rate at municipal hospitals. For example, in the years that show the largest discrepancy, 1960-62, the rate at the former was 3.9 and at the latter 0.1, or a rate that is thirty-nine times greater at the

Table 1. LEGAL ABORTIONS PER 1,000 LIVE BIRTHS

Time Period	Population	White	Nonwhite	Private Service	General Service
1952-53	New York City	4.1	1.4	3.6	1.9
1954-56	New York City	2.9	0.7	2.9	1.0
1957-59	New York City	2.8	0.6	2.4	0.6
1960-62	New York City	2.6	0.5	2.4	0.7
1960-61[a]	U.S. sample			3.17	.87
1963-65	U.S. sample	2.0	1.1		
1968	Georgia: married	0.8	0.1		
1968	Georgia: single	11.8	0.1		
1969	Georgia: married	1.2	0.4		
1969	Georgia: single	36.3	1.6		
1970 (Jan.-June)	Georgia: married	3.0	1.2		
1970 (Jan.-June)	Georgia: single	96.0	4.0		

Sources: Gold et al. (1965) for New York City; Hall (1965) and Tietze (1968) for U.S. samples; and Rochat et al. (1971) for Georgia. For details consult the original sources.

[a]These are the mean years for which data are reported from sixty major hospitals. The range of years over which data were reported is from 1951 to 1963. The rates per 1,000 live births were computed from the figures provided by Hall (1965:524-5).

private hospitals. As stated by Theodore Irwin (1970:23): "Several surveys have shown that four out of five therapeutic abortions are done on private patients—the affluent, white, and married." The affluent, white, and unmarried now also need to be included. In Table 1, we can see that the highest rates in Georgia are reported for single white women, and the largest white-black discrepancies appear for single women. In 1970, that rate was twenty-four times greater for whites than for blacks.

One possible consequence of the discrimination against the poor and against blacks in access to legal hospital abortions would be a greater turning by these groups to illegal nonhospital abortions. Although available figures on illegal abortions are understandably skimpy, the evidence that does exist suggests that the white and the affluent have also had preferential access to illegal abortions, particularly to those carried out by physicians. Lawrence Lader (1970:25-28), speaking from extensive personal knowledge of nonhospital abortions, feels that the costs and the communication networks effectively deny abortions by skilled surgeons to the poor. He notes "that far too many people are going to local midwives and hacks. Harlem Hospital receives about 400 botched abortions a year; another on the fringe of Harlem gets 250 to 300. Many never appear in abortion statistics, since staffs are humane enough to keep them from police reports if possible." Referring to Great Britain, Alice Jenkins (1961:35-36) states that their pre-reform law "presses most cruelly" on the poor who could not afford the medical care available to "the woman with knowledge, influence and financial resources." And Guttmacher (1967a:8-9) points out that "in the United States abortion is largely carried out clandestinely by physicians, particularly for the well-to-do. The poor are more likely to attempt to abort themselves or to resort to nonmedical amateurs."

One consequence of the greater reliance by the poor and blacks upon illegal abortions performed by unskilled abortionists is the higher rate of maternal mortality due to abortion. Harriet Pilpel (1967:101), discussing the situation in New York during the early 1960s, reports that 93 percent of the therapeutic abortions were performed on white private patients. She also notes that 42 percent of the pregnancy-related deaths resulted from illegal abortions and that 50 percent of these women were black, 44 percent Puerto Rican, and only 6 percent white. Her conclusion: "Even the denial of equal protection represented by segregated schools appears less heinous than this class and economic discrimination." The Gold et al. (1965:965) study of New York City from 1951 to 1962 shows that the black maternal mortality rate was about four times greater than the white rate, while the black maternal mortality rate due to abortions was about nine times the white rate, and the Puerto Rican rate was between the black and white rate. The report by Rochat et al. (1971:544) for Georgia, from 1950 to 1969, indicates a total maternal mortality rate, and an abortion-related maternal mortality rate, that are about four times higher for blacks than for whites. During the years 1965 to 1969, however, the black maternal death rate due to abortion is fourteen times the white rate. Based on national data from the National Center for Health Statistics, the black rate for abortion-related maternal mortality is 2.4 times the white rate for the years 1939-1941, 4.4 times the white rate for 1949-51, and 5.5 times the white rate for 1959-61 (Shapiro et al., 1968:148), it was 6 times the white rate in 1968 (Monthly Vital Statistics Report, 1971:7).

Gebhard and colleagues also provide information on the incidence of abortion by race and social class. They found that the percentage of pregnancies that terminate in abortion is generally higher among women at the higher educational levels, and this is especially the case among unmarried women, black and white (Gebhard et al., 1958:61, 78, 160-61). Among the married the differences between educational levels are much smaller; in fact, in the white group, the percentage of pregnancies that end in an induced abortion are somewhat higher at the lowest educational level (Gebhard et al., 1958:139, 165). In a comparison of blacks and whites, both for premarital and marital conceptions, we find that whites have higher percentages ending in induced abortions at the lower educational levels, while at the higher educational levels there is little or no difference between blacks and whites. This study, based on data that derive from interviews with women, confirms the findings of other studies reporting statistics derived from hospital records. Ignoring some variations, the data point to the greater reliance upon abortion on the part of whites over blacks, and on the part of the more affluent or more educated over the less affluent and less educated.

Changes in Access to Abortion Facilities

The large majority of the studies reporting differential abortion rates by social class or race are based upon experiences during the 1950s and the 1960s. During these years, medical indications for therapeutic abortions (to save the mother's life) were declining in importance because of medical advances, and hospital committees were being formed to make decisions about requests for abortion. These developments made it more difficult to get an abortion, and abortion rates dropped throughout most parts of the United States. During these same years, however, especially during the 1960s, the movement to incorporate social and psychological factors into the definition of health was growing, and an upsurge of interest in abortions occurred. As a result, most of the liberalized abortion laws passed between 1967 and 1970 included mental health factors as an indication for therapeutic abortions, and this led to a great deal of pressure upon psychiatrists to provide legal justification for requested abortions. The information needed to locate the most liberal hospitals and psychiatrists, the money for psychiatric consultation as well as for the abortion, and the experience needed to deal with a large array of largely white and often hostile medical personnel in order to get approval for an abortion were generally less available to black women and poor women; consequently, the abortion rate differentials between whites and blacks and between private patients and ward patients increased during the 1950s and 1960s.

During the 1950s and 1960s the abortion laws in the United States were restrictive, there was the potential of a public outcry against those who broke the laws, and enforcement was sporadic. As a result, public hospitals stuck much more closely to the letter of the abortion laws than did private hospitals. As Overstreet (1971:18) points out, abortions are desired for a great many social and economic reasons, and these "can only be approved by the subterfuge of threat to the mother's mental health." For the most part, the physician is prepared only to accommodate his own private patient, or someone that he knows on a personal basis. Typically, only private patients were likely to find physicians sufficiently interested in their welfare to bear the small risk involved in making a liberal interpretation of the abortion laws (Bell, 1971:127; Guttmacher, 1967:10 12) or in otherwise circumventing the law. Callahan (1970:139) refers to a 1967 survey by Johan Eliot reporting that more private than public hospitals accept German measles as an indication for abortion. Hall (1965:522), reporting on the year 1950 through 1960, points out that "abortions were more common among the private patients at Sloan Hospital for virtually all of the more debatable indications, such as arthritis, inactive tuberculosis, and rubella." And Kenneth R. Whittemore (1970:24) points to the substantial discrepancies between private and service patients in the number of pregnancies "accidentally" terminated as a result of a hospital D. and C. on women not listed as pregnant. In the general hospital he studied, service patients accounted for approximately half of all patients but for only about 5 percent of the lab results reporting "evidence of fetus" from D. and C.'s ostensibly performed for reasons other than terminating a pregnancy.

In brief, the evidence is rather clear that during the 1950s and 1960s the abortion rates have been higher for whites and for private patients, and that their discrepancy with rates for minority groups and public patients has increased. What about the distribution of rates by race and by social class before 1950 and after 1970? One report notes that the discrepancy was not present in Buffalo hospitals during the 1940s:

> In the 1940's, when the majority of abortions were done for
> medical reasons, the incidences on the ward and private
> services were about the same. In the 1950's, when medical
> reasons accounted for fewer abortions, the incidence on the
> private service rose to twice that of the ward service. In the
> 1960's, when the number of abortions for psychiatric or fetal
> reasons rose dramatically, the incidence on the private service
> soared to better than twenty times greater than that of the
> clinic service. (Niswander, 1967:53).

The changes in the rates that have taken place since the reform
laws of 1967, and more especially since repeal laws went into
effect in 1970, are of special interest. Although the statistics are
still fragmentary, they are perhaps a harbinger of changes to come.
Russell and Jackson (1969) report on the first full year's
experience with the liberalized abortion law in California. During
that year, 1968, the therapeutic abortion rate per 1,000 deliveries
was 7 for Medicaid patients and 14 for non-Medicaid patients;
further, county hospitals approved 71 percent of their abortion
applications in contrast to 90 percent for noncounty hospitals.
These figures, along with those reported in Table 1 for Georgia
since the liberalization of the law there, indicate that the reform
laws have not eliminated the differential rates but perhaps have
modified them. The figures for Georgia show a slight lessening of
the differential from 1968 to 1970. And Overstreet (1971:22)
feels that California has improved: "This situation is no longer
quite as discriminatory as it was before, because under the new
law hospitals involved in the care of indigent patients are doing a
fair job of carrying their share of the indicated abortions. But
economic discrimination does hit the lower middle class American
woman who is just above the level of welfare eligibility."
Theodore Irwin (1970), referring to the liberalized law in
Maryland, also feels that it has increased access of the poor to
abortions. He reports that Johns Hopkins Hospital started 1968
with about 85 percent of its therapeutic abortions for private
patients and ended the year with a 50-50 distribution. But the
most dramatic changes have taken place in those states where
repeal laws have been passed. Although pre-repeal data are not
provided, Hawaii's early experience under a repeal law indicates
that proportionately more lower income women are having

abortions than women of other income levels (Smith et al., 1971; Steinhoff et al., 1971).

In New York, based on the experience of one hospital, Strausz and Schulman (1971) noted a large increase in the percentage of blacks and Puerto Ricans receiving abortions from the first three months after the law was changed to the subsequent two months. Pakter and Nelson (1971:6-7) give abortion rate estimates for New York City residents which are comparable to those presented in Table 1 and cover the nine months subsequent to the repeal of New York's abortion laws: 422.4 for whites and 594.0 for blacks; 384.7 for private service and 525.9 for general service patients. These rates for legal abortions per 1,000 live births far exceed any of the other figures reported in Table 1 and testify to the very high demand for abortion services. The figures also indicate that the repeal law in New York has reversed the prior pattern, and now shows higher abortion rates for those groups that have higher rates of excess fertility.

The high abortion rates in New York are typical of the rates found in many other countries that have passed similar abortion laws, such as Bulgaria, Czechoslovakia, Japan, and Yugoslavia. They are also typical of the rates in several European and Latin American countries with strict abortion laws but widespread evasion. France, for example, is estimated to have as many illegal abortions as live births (Callahan, 1970:286, 289), and one survey has shown an inverse relationship between social class and abortion rates (Texier, 1969; cf. Safilios-Rothschild, 1969). It therefore appears that when abortions are readily available, either because of highly liberal legislation or widespread evasion of restrictive laws, the groups that are lower in the scale of social stratification, and presumably less successful in controlling births through contraception, are the groups that make greatest use of abortion facilities.

References

Baird, Sir Dugald. 1970. "The Obstetrician and Society." *American Journal of Public Health.* 60 (April): 628-40.

Bell, Robert R. 1971. *Social Deviance: A Substantive Analysis.* Homewood, Ill.: Dorsey, 1971.

Bogue, Donald J., ed. 1967. *Sociological Contributions to Family Planning Research.* Chicago: University of Chicago, Community and Family Study Center.

_____. 1970. *Further Sociological Contributions to Family Planning Research*. Chicago: University of Chicago, Community and Family Study Center.

_____. 1970b, Part 2. "Family Planning in the Negro Ghettos of Chicago." *Milbank Memorial Fund Quarterly* 48 (April): 283-307.

Callahan, Daniel. 1970. *Abortion: Law, Choice and Morality*. New York: Macmillan.

Campbell, Arthur A. 1968. "The Role of Family Planning in the Reduction of Poverty." *Journal of Marriage and the Family*. 30 (May): 238.

Cartwright, Ann. 1970. *Parents and Family Planning Services*. New York: Atherton.

Champion, Phyllis. 1967. "A Pilot Study of the Success or Failure of Low Income Negro Families in the Use of Birth Control." In *Sociological Contributions to Family Planning Research*, ed. Donald Bogue, pp. 112-28.

Coombs, Lolagene C., et al. 1970. "Premarital Pregnancy and Status Before and After Marriage." *American Journal of Sociology* 75 (March): 800-820.

Feldman, Joseph G., et al. 1971. "Patterns and Purposes of Oral Contraceptive Use by Economic Status." *American Journal of Public Health* 62 (June): 1089-95.

Freedman, Ronald, P.K. Whelpton, and Arthur A. Campbell. 1959. *Family Planning, Sterility and Population Growth*. New York, McGraw-Hill.

Gebhard, Paul H., et al. 1958. *Pregnancy, Birth and Abortion*. New York: Harper.

Gold, Edwin M., et al. 1965. "Therapeutic Abortions in New York City: A 20-Year Review." *American Journal of Public Health*. 55 (July): 964-72.

Guttmacher, Alan F., ed. 1967. *The Case for Legalized Abortion Now*. Berkeley: Diablo Press.

Hall, Robert. 1965. "Therapeutic Abortion, Sterilization, and Contraception." *American Journal of Obstetrics and Gynecology* 91 (February 15): 518-32.

Harrison, Colin P. 1969. "Teenage Pregnancy—Is Abortion the Answer?" *Pediatric Clinics of North America* (May), pp. 363-69.

Hill, Adelaide C. and Frederick S. Jaffe, 1967. "Negro Fertility and Family Size Preferences: Implications for Programming of Health and Social Services." In *The Negro American*, ed. Talcott Parsons and Kenneth B. Clark, pp. 205-24. Boston: Beacon.

Irwin, Theodore. March 1970. "The New Abortion Laws: How Are They Working?" *Today's Health* 48 (March): 21ff.

Jaffe, Frederic S. Jan. 1972. "Low Income Families: Fertility Changes in the 1960s." *Family Planning Perspectives* 4 (January): 43-47.

Jenkins, Alice. 1961. *Law for the Rich*. London: Victor Gollancz.

Lader, Lawrence. 1970. In *Abortion in a Changing World*, vol. 2, ed. Robert Hall. New York: Columbia University Press.

Ladner, Joyce A. 1971. *Tomorrow's Tomorrow: The Black Woman*. Garden

City, N.Y.: Doubleday.

Meier, Gitta. 1961. "The Effect of Unwanted Pregnancies on a Relief Load: An Exploratory Study." *Eugenics Quarterly* 8 (September): 142-53.

Millstone, Dorothy L. 1972. "Family Planning, Yes!... but..." *Family Planning Perspectives.* 4 (January): 20-23.

Monthly Vital Statistics Report. March 29, 1971. "Advance Report Final Mortality Statistics, 1968."

Niswander, Kenneth R. 1967. "Medical Abortion Practices in the United States." In *Abortion and the Law,* ed. David Smith, pp. 37-59. Cleveland: Press of Case Western Reserve University.

Overstreet, Edmund W. 1971. "California's Abortion Law—A Second Look." In *Abortion and the Unwanted Child,* ed. Carl Reiterman, pp. 15-26. New York: Springer.

Pakter, Jean and Frieda Nelson. 1971. "Abortion in New York City: The First Nine Months." *Family Planning Perspectives.* 3 (July): 5-12.

Pilpel, Harriet F. 1967. "The Abortion Crisis." In *The Case for Legalized Abortion Now,* ed. Alan Guttmacher, pp. 97-113.

Pohlman, Edward and Julia Mae Pohlman. 1969. *The Psychology of Birth Planning.* Cambridge, Mass.: Schenkman.

Presser, Harriet B. 1971. Part 1. "The Timing of the First Birth, Female Roles and Black Fertility." *Milbeck Memorial Fund Quarterly* 49 (July): 329-61.

Rains, Prudence Mors. 1971. *Becoming an Unwed Mother: A Sociological Account.* Chicago: Aldine, Atherton.

Rainwater, Lee. 1960. *And the Poor Get Children: Sex, Contraception, and Family Planning in the Working Class.* Chicago: Quadrangle Books.

Rochat, Roger W., Carl W. Tyler, and Albert K. Schoenbucher. 1971. "An Epidemiological Analysis of Abortion in Georgia." *American Journal of Public Health* 61 (March): 543-52.

Rodman, Hyman. 1963. "The Lower-Class Value Stretch," *Social Forces* 42 (December): Rodman et al. 1969, 205-15.

Russell, Keith P. and Edwin W. Jackson. 1969. "Therapeutic Abortions in California: First Year's Experience Under New Legislation." *American Journal of Obstetrics and Gynecology.* 105 (November 1): 757-65.

Ryan, William. 1971. *Blaming the Victim.* New York: Pantheon.

Ryder, Norman B. and Charles F. Westoff. 1971. *Reproduction in the United States 1965.* Princeton: Princeton University Press.

Safilios-Rothschild, Constantina. 1969. "Sociopsychological Factors Affecting Fertility in Urban Greece: A Preliminary Report." *Journal of Marriage and the Family.* 31 (August): 595-606.

Schulz, David A. 1969. *Coming Up Black: Patterns of Ghetto Socialization.* Englewood Cliffs, N.J.: Prentice-Hall.

Shapiro, Sam, Edward R. Schlesinger, and Robert E.L. Nesbitt, Jr. 1968. *Infant, Perinatal, Maternal, and Childhood Mortality in the United States.* Cambridge: Harvard University Press.

Smith, Roy G., et al. 1971. "Abortion in Hawaii: The First 124 Days."

American Journal of Public Health. 61 (March): 530-542.

Staples, Robert. 1972. "The Sexuality of Black Women," *Sexual Behavior* 2: 4-15.

Steinhoff, Patricia G., Roy G. Smith, and Milton Diamond. 1971. "The Characteristics and Motivations of Women Receiving Abortions." Presented at the American Sociological Association Meeting, Denver, Colorado, August 30-September 2, 1971.

Strausz, Ivan K. and Harold Schulman. 1971. "500 Outpatient Abortions Performed Under Local Anesthesia," *Obstetrics and Gynecology* 38 (August): 199-205.

Texier, Geneviève. 1969. "A Sociological Approach to Abortion" (in French). *Gynécologie practique* 20: 363-73.

Tietze, Christopher. 1968. "Therapeutic Abortions in the United States." *American Journal of Obstetrics and Gynecology* 101 (July 15): 784-87.

———. 1969. "Morality with Contraception and Induced Abortions." *Studies in Family Planning* 45 (September): 6-8.

Westoff, Leslie Aldridge and Charles F. Westoff. 1971. *From Now to Zero.* Boston: Little, Brown.

Whelpton, Pascal K., Arthur A. Campbell, and John E. Patterson. 1966. *Fertility and Family Planning in the United States.* Princeton: Princeton University Press.

Whittemore, Kenneth R. 1970. In *Abortion in a Changing World,* vol. 2, ed. Robert Hall. New York: Columbia University Press.

Zelnik, Melvin and John F. Kantner, 1970. "United States: Exploratory Studies of Negro Family Formation—Factors Relating to Illegitimacy." *Studies in Family Planning* 60 (December): 5-9.

10

How to Argue about Abortion

John T. Noonan, Jr.

At the heart of the debate about abortion is the relation of person to person in social contexts. Analogies, metaphors, and methods of debate which do not focus on persons and which do not attend to the central contexts are mischievous. Their use arises from a failure to appreciate the distinctive character of moral argument— its requirement that values be organically related and balanced, its dependence on personal vision, and its rootedness in social experience. I propose here to examine various models and methods used in the debate on abortion distinguishing those such as fantasized situations, hard cases, and linear metaphors, all of which do not work, from the balancing, seeing, and appeal to human experience which I believe to be essential. I shall move from models and metaphors which take the rule against abortion as the expression of a single value to the consideration of ways of argument intended to suggest the variety of values which have converged in the formulation of the rule. The values embodied in the rule are various because abortion is an aspect of the relation of person to person, and persons are larger than single values; and abortion is an act in a social context which cannot be reduced to a single value. I write as a critic of abortion, with no doubt a sharper eye for the weaknesses of its friends than of its foes, but my chief aim is to suggest what arguments count.

Artificial Cases

One way of reaching the nub of a moral issue is to construct a hypothetical situation endowed with precisely the characteristics you believe are crucial in the real issue you are seeking to resolve.

Isolated from the clutter of detail in the real situation, these characteristics point to the proper solution. The risk is that the features you believe crucial you will enlarge to the point of creating a caricature. The pedagogy of your illustration will be blunted by the uneasiness caused by the lack of correspondence between the fantasized situation and the real situation to be judged. Such is the case with two recent efforts by philosophers, Judith Jarvis Thomson and Michael Tooley, to construct arguments justifying abortion.

Suppose, says Thomson, a violinist whose continued existence depends on acquiring new kidneys. Without the violinist's knowledge—he remains innocent—a healthy person is kidnapped and connected to him so that the violinist now shares the use of healthy kidneys. May the victim of the kidnapping break the connection and thereby kill the violinist? Thomson intuits that the normal judgment will be Yes. The healthy person should not be imposed upon by a lifelong physical connection with the violinist. This construct, Thomson contends, bears upon abortion by establishing that being human does not carry with it a right to life which must be respected by another at the cost of serious inconvenience.[1]

This ingenious attempt to make up a parallel to pregnancy imagines a kidnapping; a serious operation performed on the victim of the kidnapping; and a continuing interference with many of the activities of the victim. It supposes that violinist and victim were unrelated. It supposes nothing by which the victim's initial aversion to his yoke-mate might be mitigated or compensated. It supposes no degree of voluntariness. The similitude to pregnancy is grotesque. It is difficult to think of another age or society in which a caricature of this sort could be seriously put forward as a paradigm illustrating the moral choice to be made by a mother.

While Thomson focuses on this fantasy, she ignores a real case from which American tort law has generalized. On a January night in Minnesota, a cattle buyer, Orlando Depue, asked a family of farmers, the Flateaus, with whom he had dined, if he could remain overnight at their house. The Flateaus refused and, although Depue was sick and had fainted, put him out of the house into the cold night. Imposing liability on the Flateaus for Depue's loss of his frostbitten fingers the court said, "In the case at bar defendants were under no contract obligation to minister to plaintiff in his distress; but humanity demanded they do so, if they understood and appreciated his condition. . . . The law as well as humanity required that he not be exposed in his helpless condition to the merciless elements."[2] Depue was a guest for supper although not a guest after supper. The American Law Institute, generalizing, has said that it makes no difference whether the helpless person is a guest or a trespasser. He has the privilege of staying. His host has the duty not to injure him or put him into an environment where he becomes nonviable. The obligation arises when one person "understands and appreciates" the condition of the other.[3] Although the analogy is not exact, the case seems closer to the mother's situation than the case imagined by Thomson; and the emotional response of the Minnesota judges seems to be a truer reflection of what humanity requires.

Michael Tooley's artificial case in defense of abortion is put forward in the course of an even broader defense by him of infanticide, horror of which he likens to other unreasoned cultural taboos. He attacks "the potentiality principle," the principle that the fetus or baby is entitled to respect because the fetus or baby will develop into an adult human being with an admitted right to life. He does so in this way. Suppose, he says, a chemical which could be injected into a kitten which would enable it to develop into a cat possessed of the brain and psychological capabilities of adult human beings. It would not be wrong, he intuits, to refrain from giving a kitten the chemical and to kill the kitten instead. Would it be wrong, he asks, to kill a kitten who had been injected? To do so would be to prevent the development of a rational adult cat. Yet, Tooley intuits, the answer must be that it would not be wrong to kill the injected kitten. Potentiality for rational adulthood, he concludes, does not enhance a kitten's claim to life, or a fetus.'[4]

Leaving the world of humans altogether, Tooley, like Thomson, has fashioned a hypothetical to give light on a very abstract question, "Who has a right to life?" The hypothetical is framed as though the subject of this question were indifferent. To get an answer we are asked to test our reactions to a fantasy. We do not have the experience to tell us what we would decide if we were confronted by his hypothetical cat or hypothetical kitten. Cat-lovers would probably respond very differently from dog-lovers. We are asked to respond to a construct, and to respond we need to see or feel the flesh and blood of a humanoid. . . .

Hard Cases and Exceptions

In the presentation of permissive abortion to the American public, major emphasis has been put on situations of great pathos—the child deformed by thalidomide, the child affected by rubella, the child known to suffer from Tay-Sachs disease or Downs syndrome, the raped adolescent, the exhausted mother of small children. These situations are not imagined, and the cases described are not analogies to those where abortion might be sought; they are themselves cases to which abortion is a solution. Who could deny the poignancy of their appeal?

Hard cases make bad law, runs the venerable legal adage, but it seems to be worse law if the distress experienced in situations such as these is not taken into account. If persons are to be given preeminence over abstract principle, should not exceptions for these cases be made in the most rigid rule against abortion? Does not the human experience of such exceptions point to a more sweeping conclusion—the necessity of abandoning any uniform prohibition of abortion, so that all the elements of a particular situation may be weighted by the woman in question and her doctor?

So far, fault can scarcely be found with this method of argumentation, this appeal to common experience. But the cases are oversimplified if focus is directed solely on the parents of a physically defective child or on the mother in the cases of rape or psychic exhaustion. The situations are very hard for the parents or the mother; they are still harder for the fetus who is threatened with death. If the fetus is a person as the opponents of abortion contend, its destruction is not the sparing of suffering by the sacrifice of a principle but by the sacrifice of a life. Emotion is a proper element in moral response, but to the extent that the emotion generated by these cases obscures the claims of the fetus, this kind of argumentation fosters erroneous judgment.

In three of the cases—the child deformed by drugs, disease, or genetic defect—the neglect of the child's point of view seems stained by hypocrisy. Abortion is here justified as putting the child out of the misery of living a less than normal life. The child is not consulted as to the choice. Experience, which teaches that even the most seriously incapacitated prefer living to dying, is ignored. The feelings of the parents are the actual consideration, and these feelings are treated with greater tenderness than the fetal desire to live. The common unwillingness to say frankly that the abortion is sought for the parents' benefit is testimony, unwillingly given, to the intuition that such self-preference by the parents is difficult for society or for the parents themselves to accept.

The other kind of hard case does not mask preference for the parent by a pretense of concern for the fetus. The simplest situation is that of a pregnancy due to rape—in presentations to some legislatures it was usual to add a racist fillip by supposing a white woman and a black rapist—but this gratuitous pandering to bias is not essential. The fetus, unwanted in the most unequivocal way, is analogized to an invader of the mother's body—is it even appropriate to call her a mother when she did nothing to assume the special fiduciary cares of motherhood? If she is prevented from having an abortion, she is being compelled for nine months to be reminded of a traumatic assault. Do not her feelings override the right to life of her unwanted tenant?

Rape arouses fear and a desire for revenge, and reference to rape evokes emotion. The emotion has been enough for the state to take the life of the rapist.[5] Horror of the crime is easily extended to horror of the product, so that the fetal life becomes forfeit too. If horror is overcome, adoption appears to be a more humane solution than abortion. If the rape case is not being used as a stalking horse by proponents of abortion—if there is a desire to deal with it in itself—the solution is to assure the destruction of the sperm in the one to three days elapsing between insemination and impregnation.

Generally, however, the rape case is presented as a way of suggesting a general principle, a principle which could be formulated as follows: Every unintended pregnancy may be interrupted if its continuation will cause emotional distress to the mother. Pregnancies due to bad planning or bad luck are analogized to pregnancies due to rape; they are all involuntary.[6] Indeed many pregnancies can without great difficulty be assimilated to the hard case, for how often do persons undertake an act of sexual intercourse consciously intending that a child be the fruit of that act? Many pregnancies are unspecified by a particular intent, are unplanned, are in this sense involuntary. Many pregnancies become open to termination if only the baby consciously sought has immunity.

This result is unacceptable to those who believe that the fetus is human. It is acceptable to those who do not believe the fetus is human, but to reach it they do not need the argument based on the hard case. The result would follow immediately from the mother's dominion over a portion of her body. Opponents of abortion who out of consideration for the emotional distress caused by rape will grant the rape exception must see that the exception can be generalized to destroy the rule. If, on other grounds they believe the rule good, they must deny the exception which eats it up.

Direct and Indirect

From paradigmatic arguments, I turn to metaphors and especially those which, based on some spatial image, are misleading. I shall begin with "direct" and "indirect" and their cousins, "affirmative" and "negative." In the abortion argument "direct" and "indirect," "affirmative" and "negative" occur more frequently in these kinds of questions: If one denies that a fetus may be killed directly, but admits that indirect abortion is permissible, is he guilty of inconsistency? If one maintains that there is a negative duty not to kill fetuses, does he thereby commit himself to an affirmative obligation of assuring the safe delivery of every fetus? If one agrees that there is no affirmative duty to actualize as many spermatic, ovoid, embryonic, or fetal potentialities as possible, does one thereby concede that it is generally permissible to take steps to destroy fertilized ova? The argumentative implications of these questions can be best unravelled by looking at the force of the metaphors invoked.

"Direct" and "indirect" appeal to our experience of linedrawing and of travel. You reach a place on a piece of paper by drawing a straight or crooked line—the line is direct or indirect. You go to a place without detours or you go in a roundabout fashion—your route is direct or indirect. In each instance, whether your path is direct or indirect your destination is the same. The root experience is that you can reach the same spot in ways distinguished by their immediacy and the amount of ground covered. "Indirectly" says you proceed more circuitously and cover more ground. It does not, however, say anything of the reason why you go circuitously. You may go indirectly because you want to cover more ground or because you want to disguise your destination.

The ambiguity in the reason for indirectness—an ambiguity present in the primary usage of the term—carries over when "indirect" is applied metaphorically to human intentions. There may be a reason for doing something indirectly—you want to achieve another objective besides the indirect action. You may also act indirectly to conceal from another or from yourself what is your true destination. Because of this ambiguity in the reason for indirection, "indirect" is apt to cause confusion when applied in moral analysis.

Defenders of an absolute prohibition of abortion have excepted the removal of a fertilized ovum in an ectopic pregnancy and the removal of a cancerous uterus containing an embryo. They have characterized the abortion involved as "indirect." They have meant that the surgeon's attention is focused on correcting a pathological condition dangerous to the mother and he only performs the operation because there is no alternative way of correcting it.[7] But the physician has to intend to achieve not only the improvement of the mother but the performance of action by which the fertilized ovum becomes nonviable. He necessarily intends to perform an abortion, he necessarily intends to kill. To say that he acts indirectly is to conceal what is being done. It is a confusing and improper use of the metaphor.[8]

A clearer presentation of the cases of the cancerous uterus and the ectopic pregnancy would acknowledge them to be true exceptions to the absolute inviolability of the fetus. Why are they not exceptions which would eat up the rule? It depends on what the rule is considered to be. The principle that can be discerned in them is, whenever the embryo is a danger to the life of the mother, an abortion is permissible. At the level of reason nothing more can be asked of the mother. The exceptions do eat up any rule of preferring the fetus to the mother—any rule of fetus first. They do not destroy the rule that the life of the fetus has precedence over other interests of the mother. The exceptions of the ectopic pregnancy and the cancerous uterus are special cases of the general exception to the rule against killing, which permits one to kill in self-defense. Characterization of this kind of killing as "indirect" does not aid analysis.[9]

It is a basic intuition that one is not responsible for all the consequences of one's acts. By living at all one excludes others from the air one breathes, the food one eats. One cannot foresee all the results which will flow from any given action. It is imperative for moral discourse to be able to distinguish between injury foreseeably inflicted on another, and the harm which one may unknowingly bring about. "Direct" and "indirect" are sometimes used to distinguish the foreseen consequences from the unconsidered or unknown consequence. This usage does not justify terming abortion to save a mother's life "indirect." In the case of terminating the ectopic pregnancy, the cancerous uterus, the life-threatening fetus generally, one considers precisely the consequence, the taking of the fetal life.

Just as one intuits that one is not responsible for all the consequences, so one intuits that one is not called to right all wrongs. No one is bound to the impossible. There is, therefore, an intuitive difference between the duty to refrain from doing harm to anyone and the duty to help everyone in distress. The duty to refrain is possible of fulfillment if it refers only to conscious infliction of harm. The duty to help is impossible if one is going to develop as a human being, getting educated, earning a living, marrying, raising a family, and so forth. The needs of other human beings are subordinated or postponed by everyone to the fulfillment of many of one's own needs, and rightly so. The distinction between affirmative and negative duties, another linear metaphor, rests on this universal experience. The terms do have a basis in moral life. Their usefulness in moral analysis, however, is not great. The crucial distinction is not between negative and affirmative, but between limited and unlimited duty.

It is possible to state the duty not to kill the fetus as the duty to care for the fetus. Opponents of abortion, however, do not commit thereby themselves to the position that all fertilized ova must be born. A pregnant woman may, for example, take the chance of killing the baby by going for a walk or a drive instead of staying safely in bed. She is not responsible for all the consequences of her acts. She is not called to help the fetus in every possible way. The negative duty or the convertible affirmative duty excludes acts which have a high probability of death for the fetus, but not those with a low probability of death. Similarly, one has a duty not to kill one's older children, and a duty to care for them, but no duty to keep them free from all risk of harm. No inconsistency exists in not equating a limited negative duty with an unlimited affirmative duty; no inconsistency exists in rejecting high risk acts and approving low risks acts.[10]

Linedrawing

The prime linear metaphor is, of course, linedrawing. It is late in the history of moral thought for anyone to suppose that an effective moral retort is, "Yes, but where do you draw the line?" or to make the inference that, because any drawing of a line requires a decision, all linedrawing is arbitrary. One variant or another of these old ploys is, however, frequently used in the present controversy. From living cell to dying corpse a continuum exists. Proponents of abortion are said to be committed to murder, to euthanasia, or, at a minimum, to infanticide. Opponents are alleged to be bound to condemn contraception—after all, spermatazoa are living human cells. Even if contraception is admitted and infanticide rejected, the range of choice is still large enough for the line drawn to be challenged—is it to be at nidation, at formation of the embryo, at quickening, at viability, at birth? Whoever adopts one point is asked why he does not move forward or backward by one stage of development. The difficulty of presenting apodictic reasons for preferring one position is made to serve as proof that the choice may be made as best suits the convenience of an individual or the state.[11]

The metaphor of linedrawing distracts attention from the nature of the moral decision. The metaphor suggests an empty room composed of indistinguishable grey blocks. In whatever way the room is divided, there are grey blocks on either side of the line. Or if the metaphor is taken more mathematically, it suggests a series of points, which, wherever bisected, are fungible with each other. What is obscured in the spatial or mathematical model is the variety of values whose comparison enters into any moral decision. The model appeals chiefly to those novices in moral reasoning who believe that moral judgment is a matter of pursuing a principle to its logical limit. Single-mindedly looking at a single value, they ask, if this is good, why not more of it? In practice, however, no one can be so single-hearted. Insistence of this kind of logical consistency becomes the preserve of fanatics or of controversialists eager to convict their adversaries of inconsistency. If more than one good is sought by a human being, he must bring the goods he seeks into relationship with each other; he must limit one to maintain another; he must mix them.[12]

The process of choosing multiple goods occurs in many particular contexts—in eating, in studying, in painting. No one supposes that those who take the first course must forego dessert, that the election of English means History shall not be studied, that the use of blue excludes red. Linear models for understanding choice in these matters are readily perceived as inappropriate. The commitment to values, the cutting off of values, and the mixing of values accompany each other.

Is, however, the choice of the stage of development which should not be destroyed by abortion a choice requiring the mixing of multiple goods? Is not the linear model appropriate when picking a point on the continuum of life? Are not the moral choices which require commitment and mixing made only after the selection of the stage at which a being becomes a person? To these related questions the answers must all be negative. To recognize a person is a moral decision; it depends on objective data but it also depends on the perceptions and inclinations and ends of the decision makers; it cannot be made without commitment and without consideration of alternative values. Who is a person? This is not a question asked abstractly, in the air, with no purpose in mind. To disguise the personal involvement in the response to personhood is to misconceive the issue of abortion from the start.

Those who identify the rational with the geometrical, the algebraic, the logical may insist that, if the fundamental recognition of personhood depends upon the person who asks, then the arbitrariness of any position on abortion is conceded. If values must be mixed even in identifying the human, who can object to another's mixture? The issue becomes like decisions in eating, studying, and painting, a matter of discretion. A narrow rationalism of this kind uses "taste" as the ultimate epithet for the nonrational. It does not acknowledge that each art has its own rules. It claims for itself alone the honorable term "reason."

As this sort of monopoly has become unacceptable in general philosophy, so it is unnecessary to accept it here. Taste, that is perceptiveness, is basic; and if it cannot be disputed, it can be improved by experience. Enology, painting, or moral reasoning all require basic aptitude, afford wide ranges of options, have limits beyond which a choice can be counterproductive, and are better done by the experienced than by amateurs. Some persons may lack almost any capacity for undertaking one or another of them. Although all men are moral beings, not all are proficient at moral judgment, so that morality is not a democratic business. Selecting multiple goods, those who are capable of the art perceive, test, mix and judge. The process has little in common with linedrawing. In the case of abortion, it is the contention of its opponents that in such a process the right response to the data is that the fetus is a human being.[13]

Balancing

The process of decisionmaking just described is better caught by the term "balancing." In contrast to linedrawing, balancing is a metaphor helpful in understanding moral judgment. Biologically understood, balancing is the fundamental metaphor for moral reasoning. A biological system is in balance when its parts are in the equilibrium necessary for it to live. To achieve such equilibrium, some parts—the heart, for example—must be preserved at all costs; others may be sacrificed to maintain the whole. Balance in the biological sense does not demand an egalitarian concern for every part, but an ordering and subordination which permit the whole to function. So in moral reasoning the reasoner balances values.

The mistaken common reading of this metaphor is to treat it as equivalent to weighing, so that balancing is understood as an act of quantitative comparison analogous to that performed by an assayer or a butcher. This view tacitly supposes that values are weights which are tangible and commensurate. One puts so many units on one pan of the scales and matches them with so many units on the other to reach a "balanced" judgment. To give a personal example, Daniel Callahan has questioned my position that the value of innocent life cannot be sacrificed to achieve the other values which abortion might secure. The "force of the rule," he writes, "is absolutist, displaying no 'balance' at all."[14] He takes balancing in the sense of weighing and wonders how one value can be so heavy.

That justice often consists in the fair distribution or exchange of goods as in the familiar Aristotelian examples has no doubt worked to confirm a quantitative approach. Scales as the symbol of justice seem to suggest the antiquity of the quantitative meaning of balance. But the original sense of the scales was otherwise. In Egypt where the symbol was first used, a feather, the Egyptian hieroglyphic for truth, turned the balance. As put by David Daube in his illuminating analysis of the ancient symbolism, "The slightest turning of the scales—'but in the estimation of a hair'—will decide the issue, and the choice is between salvation and annihilation."[15] Not a matching of weights, but a response to reality was what justice was seen to require, and what was at stake was not a slight overweighing in one direction or the other, but salvation. Moral choice, generally, has this character of a hair separating good from evil.

A fortiori then, in moral judgment, where more values are in play than in any system of strict law or commutative justice, balancing is a misleading metaphor if it suggests a matching of weights. It is an indispensable metaphor if it stands for the equilibrium of a living organism making the choices necessary for its preservation. A single value cannot be pursued to the point of excluding all other values. This is the caricature of moral argument I have already touched on in connection with the metaphor of linedrawing. But some values are more vital than others, as the heart is more vital to the body than the hand. A balanced moral judgment requires a sense of the limits, interrelations, and priority of values. It is the position of those generally opposed to abortion that a judgment preferring interests less than human life to human life is unbalanced, that a judgment denying a mother's fiduciary responsibility to her child is unbalanced, that a judgment making killing a principal part of the profession of a physician is unbalanced, that a judgment permitting agencies of the state to procure and pay for the destruction of the offspring of the poor or underprivileged is unbalanced. They contend that such judgments expand the right limits of a mother's responsibility for herself, destroy the fiduciary relation which is a central paradigm for the social bond, fail to relate to the physician's service to life and the state's care for its citizens. At stake in the acceptance of abortion is not a single value, life, against which the suffering of the mother or parents may be balanced. The values to be considered are the child's life, the mother's faithfulness to her dependent, the physician's commitment to preserving life; and in the United States today abortion cannot be discussed without awareness that if law does not prohibit it, the state will fund it, so that the value of the state's abstention from the taking of life is also at issue. The judgment which accepts abortion, it is contended, is unbalanced in subordinating these values to the personal autonomy of the mother and the social interest in population control.

Seeing

The metaphor of balancing points to the process of combining values. But we do not combine values like watercolors. We respond to values situated in subjects. "Balancing" is an inadequate metaphor for moral thinking in leaving out of account the central moral transaction—the response of human beings to other human beings.[16] In making moral judgments we respond to those human beings whom we see.

The metaphor of sight is a way of emphasizing the need for perception, whether by eyes or ears or touch, of those we take as subjects to whom we respond. Seeing in any case is more than the registration of a surface. It is a penetration yielding some sense of the other's structure, so that the experiencing of another is never merely visual or auditory or tactile. We see the features and comprehend the humanity at the same time. Look at the fetus, say the anti-abortionists, and you will see humanity. How long, they ask, can a man turn his head and pretend that he just doesn't see?

An accusation of blindness, however, does not seem to advance moral argument. A claim to see where others do not see is a usual claim of charlatans. "Illumination" or "enlightenment" appear to transcend experience and make moral disputation impossible. "Visionary" is often properly a term of disparagement. Is not an appeal to sight the end of rational debate?

In morals, as in epistemology, there is nonetheless no substitute for perception. Are animals within the range of beings with a right to life, and babies not, as Michael Tooley has recently suggested? Should trees be persons, as Christopher Stone has recently maintained?[17] Questions of this kind are fundamentally frivolous for they point to the possibility of moral argument while attempting to deny the foundation of moral argument, our ability to recognize human persons. If a person could in no way perceive another person to be like himself, he would be incapable of moral response. If a person cannot perceive a cat or a tree as different from himself, he cuts off the possibility of argument. Debate should not end with pointing, but it must begin there.

Is there a contradiction in the opponents of abortion appealing to perception when fetuses are normally invisible? Should one not hold that until beings are seen they have not entered the ranks of society? Falling below the threshold of sight, do not fetuses fall below the threshold of humanity? If the central moral transaction is response to the other person, are not fetuses peculiarly weak subjects to elicit our response? These questions pinpoint the principal task of the defenders of the fetus—to make the fetus visible. The task is different only in degree from that assumed by defenders of other persons who have been or are "overlooked." For centuries, color acted as a psychological block to perception, and the blindness induced by color provided a sturdy basis for discrimination. Minorities of various kinds exist today who are "invisible" and therefore unlikely to be "heard" in the democratic process. Persons literally out of sight of society in prisons and mental institutions are often not "recognized" as fellow humans by the world with which they have "lost touch." In each of these instances those who seek to vindicate the rights of the unseen must begin by calling attention to their existence. "Look" is the exhortation they address to the callous and the negligent.[18]

Perception of fetuses is possible with not substantially greater effort than that required to pierce the physical or psychological barriers to recognizing other human beings. The main difficulty is everyone's reluctance to accept the extra burdens of care imposed by an expansion of the numbers in whom humanity is recognized. It is generally more convenient to have to consider only one's kin, one's peers, one's country, one's race. Seeing requires personal attention and personal response. The emotion generated by identification with a human form is necessary to overcome the inertia which is protected by a vision restricted to a convenient group. If one is willing to undertake the risk that more will be required in one's action, fetuses may be seen in multiple ways—circumstantially, by the observation of a pregnant woman; photographically, by pictures of life in the womb; scientifically, in accounts written by investigators of prenatal life and child psychologists; visually, by observing a blood transfusion or an abortion while the fetus is alive or by examination of a fetal corpse after death.[19] The proponent of abortion is invited to consider the organism kicking the mother, swimming peacefully in amniotic fluid, responding to the prick of an instrument, being extracted from the womb, sleeping in death. Is the kicker or swimmer similar to him or to her? Is the response to pain like his or hers? Will his or her own face look much different in death?

Response

Response to the fetus begins with grasp of the data which yield the fetus' structure. That structure is not merely anatomical form;

it is dynamic—we apprehend the fetus' origin and end. It is this apprehension which makes response to the nameless fetus different from the conscious analogizing that goes on when we name a cat. Seeing, we are linked to the being in the womb by more than an inventory of shared physical characteristics and by more than a number of made-up psychological characteristics. The weakness of the being as potential recalls our own potential state, the helplessness of the being evokes the human condition of contingency. We meet another human subject.

Seeing is impossible apart from experience, but experience is the most imprecise of terms. What kind of experience counts, and whose? There are experiences which only women and usually only those within the ages of 14 to 46 who are fertile can have: conceiving a child, carrying a child, having an abortion, being denied an abortion, giving birth. There are experiences only a fetus can have: being carried, being aborted, being born. There is the experience of obstetricians who regularly deliver children and occasionally abort them; there is the differently textured experience of the professional abortionist. There is the experience of nurses who prepare the mother for abortion, care for her after the abortion, and dispose of the aborted fetus. There is the experience of physicians, social workers, and ministers, who advise a woman to have an abortion or not to have one. There is the experience of those who enforce a law against abortion, and those who stealthily or openly, for profit or for conscience's sake, defy it. There is the experience of those who have sexual intercourse knowing that abortion is or is not a remedy if an accidental pregnancy should result. There is the experience of society at large of a pattern of uncontrolled abortion or of its regulation.

Some arguments are unduly exclusivist in the experience they will admit. Those who suggest that abortion is peculiarly a matter for women disqualify men because the unique experience of pregnancy is beyond their achievement. Yet such champions of abortion do not regularly disqualify sterile women whose experience of pregnancy must be as vicarious as a man's. Tertullian taught that only those who have known motherhood themselves have a right to speak from experience on the choices presented by abortion.[20] Yet even Tertullian did not go so far as to say that only mothers who had both given birth and had had abortions were qualified to speak. Efforts of this sort to restrict those who are competent rest on a confusion between the relevant and the personal. You do not have to be a judge to know that bribery is evil or a slave to know that slavery is wrong. Vicarious experience, in this as in other moral matters, is a proper basis for judgment.

Vicarious experience appears strained to the outer limit when one is asked to consider the experience of the fetus. No one remembers being born, no one knows what it is like to die. Empathy may, however, supply for memory, as it does in other instances when we refer to the experience of infants who cannot speak or to the experience of death by those who cannot speak again. The experience of the fetus is no more beyond our knowledge than the experience of the baby and the experience of the dying.

Participation in an abortion is another sort of experience relevant to moral judgment. Generals are not thought of as the best judges of the morality of war, nor is their experience thought to be unaffected by their profession, but they should be heard, when the permissibility of war is urged. Obstetricians are in an analogous position, their testimony subject to a discount. The testimony of professional abortionists is also relevant, although subject to an even greater discount. Nurses are normally more disinterested witnesses. They speak as ones who have empathized with the female patient, disposed of the fetal remains, and, like the Red Cross in wartime, have known what the action meant by seeing the immediate consequences.

The experience of individuals becomes a datum of argument through autobiography and testimony, inference and empathy. The experience of a society has to be captured by the effort of sociologists and novelists, historians and lawyers, psychologists and moralists; and it is strongly affected by the prism of the medium used. Typically the proponents of abortion have put emphasis on quantitative evidence—for example, on the number of abortions performed in the United States or in the world at large. The assumption underlying this appeal to experience is that what is done by a great many persons cannot be bad, is indeed normal. This assumption, often employed when sexual behavior is studied, is rarely favored when racial discrimination or war are considered. It is a species of natural law, identifying the usual with the natural. The experience appealed to counts as argument only for those who accept this identification and consider the usual the good.

Psychological evidence has been called upon by the opponents of abortion. Trauma and guilt have been found associated with the election of abortion. The inference is made that abortion is the cause of this unhappiness. As in many arguments based on social consequences, however, the difficulty is to isolate the cause. Do persons undergoing abortion have character predispositions which would in any event manifest themselves in psychic disturbance? Do they react as they do because of social conditioning which could be changed to encourage a positive attitude to abortion? Is the act of abortion at the root of their problems or the way in which the process is carried out? None of these questions is settled; the evidence is most likely to be convincing to those already inclined to believe that abortion is an evil.[21]

Another kind of experience is that embedded in law. In Roman law where children generally had little status independent of their parents, the fetus was "a portion of the mother or her viscera." This view persisted in nineteenth-century American tort law, Justice Holmes in a leading case describing the fetus as "a part of the body of the mother." In recent years, however, the tort cases have asked, in Justice Bok's phrase, if the fetus is a person; and many courts have replied affirmatively. The change, a striking revolution in torts law, came from the courts incorporating into their thought new biological data on the fetus as a living organism.[22] Evidence on how the fetus is now perceived is also provided by another kind of case where abortion itself is not involved—the interpretation in wills and trusts of gifts to "children" or "issue." In these cases a basic question is, "What is the common understanding of people when they speak of children?" The answer, given repeatedly by American courts, is that "the average testator" speaking of children means to include a being who has been conceived but not born.[23] Free from the distorting pressures of the conflict over abortion, this evidence of the common understanding suggests that social experience has found the fetus to be within the family of man.

The most powerful expression of common experience is that given by art and literature. Birth has almost everywhere been celebrated in painting. The Nativity has been a symbol of gladness not only because of its sacral significance, but because of its human meaning—"joy that a man is born into the world." Abortion, in contrast, has rarely been the subject of art. Unlike other forms of death, abortion has not been seen by painters as a release, a sacrifice, or a victory. Characteristically it has stood for sterility, futility, and absurdity. Consider, for example, Orozco's mural, "Gods of the Modern World" in the Baker Library at

Dartmouth College.[24] Academia is savagely satirized by portraying professors as impotent attendants in an operating room in which truth is stillborn. Bottled fetuses in the foreground attest the professors' habitual failure. The entire force of the criticism of academic achievement comes from the painter's knowledge that everyone will recognize abortion as a grave defeat and the bottling of dead fetuses as a travesty of healthy birth. Whoever sees such a painting sees how mankind has commonly experienced abortion.

In contemporary American literature, John Updike's *Couples* comments directly upon abortion, using it at a crucial turn as both event and symbol. Piet Hanema, married to Angela, has promiscuously pursued other married women, among them Foxy Whitman, who is now pregnant by him. They have this exchange:

> "All I know is what *I* honestly want. I want this damn thing to stop growing inside me."
> "Don't cry."
> "Nature is *so* stupid. It has all my maternal glands working, do you know what that means, Piet? You know what the great thing about being pregnant I found out was? It's something I just couldn't have imagined. You're never alone. When you have a baby inside you you are not alone. It's a person."[25]

To procure the abortion it becomes necessary for Piet to surrender his own wife Angela to Freddy, who has access to the abortionist. Embarked upon his course Piet does not stop at this act which destroys his own marriage irretrievably. Foxy's feelings at the time of the abortion are then described through Piet:

> Not until days later, after Foxy had survived the forty-eight hours alone in the house with Toby and the test of Ken's return from Chicago, did Piet learn, not from Freddy but from her as told by Freddy, that at the moment of anesthesia she had panicked; she had tried to strike the Negress pressing the sweet, sweet mask to her face and through the first waves of ether had continued to cry that she should go home, that she was supposed to have this baby, that the child's father was coming to smash the door down with a hammer and would stop them.[26]

Updike's only comment as an author is given as Piet then goes to Foxy's house: "Death, once invited in, leaves his muddy bootprints everywhere."[27] The elements of the experience of abortion are here: the hatred of the depersonalized burden growing, willy-nilly, in the womb; the sense of a baby, a person, one's own child; the desperate desire to be rid of the burden extinguishing all other considerations; the ineffectual hope of delivery the moment before the child's death. A mask covers the human face of the mother. Symbolically the abortion seals a course of infidelity. Conclusively it becomes death personified.

The Experience of Christians

Ethics generally or Christian ethics specifically do not exist in the fashion of some impersonal science, so that one can say with professorial pomposity, "Ethics teaches." Ethics exists in particular men and women formulating rules and sharing values within particular communities. For the Christian, vicarious experience of special significance is the experience of the religious community of which he or she is a part. Reference to that experience distinguishes the ethics done by Christians from the ethics done by Hindus or humanists. No one makes up an ethical position out of whole cloth. Everyone speaks from inside an environment.[28] The Christian speaks not only from a vantage point in a civil society, but as a member of an ecclesial community which is both contemporary and historical. It is in this sense that there is an experience which Christians share and, consequent on it, an ethics done by Christians. The experience of Christians does not cancel other social experience. A Christian forming an ethical position cannot ignore other social experience. He or she incorporates such experience with the experience of Christians in formulating a response.

Since a time contemporaneous with the composition of the Gospels, the teaching of Christians has been that abortion is a denial of human love and the destruction of a being created in the image of God. In nineteen centuries of Christian life, the social discipline enforcing the teaching has varied and the possibility of exceptions to it has been explored. The teaching itself has remained firm. At one level the teaching appears impersonal—the assertion of a rule. But the rule protects values of life, responsibility and love located in persons, and these values are what the Christian community has held dear in responding to human persons in the light of the Christian's imitation of Christ. The rule against abortion is founded on the experience of Christians. It was formed early, maintained for several centuries in a hostile society, then reflected in the law of professedly Christian nations, and accepted in each generation by the community of believers as embodying the requirements of the love of neighbor and of God.[29]

To be uninterested in the history of this Christian conviction is perhaps an unexceptionable stand for a non-Christian; for a Christian it is to disavow the community in time. New moral insights, as experience changes and consciousness develops, are always possible and welcome. But to be genuine development, such insights must take into account the response of the community in the past. To ignore the earlier response is to cut oneself off from the community as it has historically existed. As members of this community, we are called to respond to persons today taking seriously the values of persons in the past.

This response to the community is integrally linked for the Christian to faith. His or her own experience living as a Christian person is to be taken into account. The Christian person responds to the persons, the friends, who are encountered. At the center of the circle of friends, past and present, to whom the Christian responds, is Jesus, so that our response is not to dead history—let the dead bury the dead—but to one who has called us as likenesses and friends.

Notes

1. Judith Thomson, "A Defense of Abortion," *Philosophy & Public Affairs* 1 (Princeton, N.J.: Princeton University Press, 1972), pp. 48-49, 55-56.

2. *Depue v. Flateau* 100 Minn. 299, 111 W.W. 1 (1907).

3. American Law Institute, *Restatement of Torts, Second* (1965) sec. 197.

4. Michael Tooley, "Abortion and Infanticide," *Philosophy & Public Affairs* 2 (Princeton, N.J.: Princeton University Press, 1973), pp. 60-62.

5. See Note, "Constitutional Law: Capital Punishment for Rape Constitutes Cruel and Unusual Punishment When No Life is Taken or Endangered," *Minnesota Law Review* 95 (1971), p. 56.

6. See Thomson, op. cit.,"A Defense of Abortion," p. 59.

7. See my "An Almost Absolute Value in History," Noonan, ed., *The Morality of Abortion* (Cambridge, Mass.: Harvard University Press, 1970), pp. 46-50.

8. To say that the act is in itself good seems to me to be an impossible

supposition—there is no human act "in itself" apart from intent. See, for a contrary analysis, Germain Grisez, *Abortion: The Myths, The Realities, and the Arguments* (Washington: Corpus Books, 1970), p. 329.

9. For a comparable analysis of the use of direct and indirect in constitutional law, see D. J. Farage, "That Which 'Directly' Affects Interstate Commerce," *Dickinson Law Review* 42 (Carlisle, Pa.: Dickinson Law School, 1937), p. 71.

10. For analysis of affirmative and negative duties in tort law, see John G. Fleming, *The Law of Torts* (Sydney: Law Book Co., 2 ed., 1961), pp. 148-51.

11. Even Roger Wertheimer, who has made a good explication of the anti-abortion argument from the point of view of one who does not accept it, ends his article by a question-begging device—the burden of proof of fetal humanity, he says, is on the state. Wertheimer, "Understanding the Abortion Argument," *Philosophy & Public Affairs* 1 (op. cit. 1971), pp. 94-95. From the viewpoint of opponents of abortion, his argument may be reshaped: the state has the burden of proving that its actions are legitimate; laws which permit the killing of the fetus seriously threaten human life; they may be sustained only if the state can show that the fetus is not human; and this cannot be done.

12. For an example of the controversialist's use of linedrawing, see Glanville Williams, *The Sanctity of Life and the Criminal Law* (New York: Knopf, 1957), p. 704. For an approach which does not recognize that values must be cut off—that insists we must be "open" to basic values, see Grisez, *Abortion: The Myths, the Realities, and the Arguments* (op. cit.), pp. 310-21. Grisez is followed by John Finnis, "The Rights and Wrongs of Abortion," *Philosophy & Public Affairs* 2 (op. cit., 1973), p. 126.

13. E.g., my article, "Deciding Who is Human," *Natural Law Forum* 12 (South Bend, Ind: Notre Dame School of Law, 1968), pp. 134-40.

14. Daniel Callahan, *Abortion: Law, Choice, and Morality* (New York: Macmillan, 1970), pp. 430-31.

15. David Daube, "The Scales of Justice," *Juridical Review* 63 (So. Hackensack, N.J.: Rothman, 1951), p. 113.

16. See Enda McDonagh, "The Structure and the Basis of the Moral Experience," *Irish Theological Quarterly* 38:1 (Maynooth, Ireland: St. Patrick's College, 1971), pp. 3-20.

17. Michael Tooley, "Abortion and Infanticide," pp. 64-65; Christopher Stone, "Should Trees Have Standing? Toward Legal Rights for Natural Objects," *Southern California Law Review*, 45 (Los Angeles: Univ. So. Calif., 1972) pp. 450-501. The same position on trees is taken by Justice William O. Douglas, dissenting, in *Sierra Club v. Morton*, 405 (U.S. Reports (1972), p. 727.

18. On our complaisance if we cannot see mutilations or the mutilated, David Daube, *Legal Problems in Medical Advance* (Jerusalem, 1971), pp. 19-22. See also the extensive treatment of the meaning of touch in Ashley

Montague, *Touching* (New York: Columbia, 1972).

19. See, e.g., Beth Day and H.M.I. Liley, *Modern Motherhood: Pregnancy, Childbirth, and the Newborn Baby* (1967 ed.), pp. 23-24, 30-31. In the brief the state in *Doe v. Wade,* Supreme Court of the United States, October Term, 1970, number 980, possibly the most effective argument was the photograph of an outstretched fetal hand; it was recognizably a human hand.

20. Tertullian, *De anima* (ed. J. H. Wasink, 1947), 25.5.

21. See Callahan, *Abortion: Law, Choice and Morality,* (op. cit.), pp. 67-71.

22. On this development, see Noonan, ed., *The Morality of Abortion* (op. cit.), pp. 6-7, 226-230; William Prosser, *Handbook of the Law of Torts* (St. Paul: West, 3d ed., 1964), sec. 56; Edwin W. Patterson, *Law in a Scientific Age* (New York: Columbia, 1963), p. 65.

23. A. James Casner, ed., *American Law of Property* (Boston: Little, Brown, 1952), vol. 7, sec. 22.3; 249; sec. 22, 42, 358.

24. Reproduced in *The Orozco Frescoes at Dartmouth* (Dartmouth College, 1934).

25. *Couples* (New York: Knopf, 1968), p. 360.

26. Ibid., pp. 378-79.

27. Ibid., p. 380.

28. Cf. Josef Fuchs, S.J., "The Absoluteness of Moral Terms," *Gregorianum* 52 (Rome: Pontificia Universita Gregoriana, 1971). p. 453.

29. On this history, see my "An Almost Absolute Value in History," Noonan, ed., *The Morality of Abortion* (op. cit.), pp. 8-50.

11

The Abortion Culture

Nick Thimmesch

A journalist often gets caught up in events flaring into instant print and broadcast—a Watergate, feverish inflation, a fretful fuel crisis. We grab at these, try to make some sense out of it all and soon turn to what's next. Occasionally we come on to something that strikes the core and won't go away. For me, it has been the question of the value of human life—a question embracing abortion, letting the newborn die, euthanasia and the creeping utilitarian ethic in medicine that impinges on human dignity. It's all reminiscent of the "what is useful is good" philosophy of German medicine in the '30s—a utilitarianism that sent 275,000 "unworthy" Germans to death and helped bring on the Hitler slaughter of millions of human beings a few years later.

Now super-abortionists and others who relish monkeying around with human life cry that this is scare stuff inspired by hysterical Catholics waving picket signs. Not so. There is growing concern among Protestant and Jewish thinkers about "right to life" and the abortion-binge mentality.

Fetal life has become cheap. There were an estimated 1,340,000 legal and illegal abortions in the U.S. last year. There were a whopping 540,245 abortions in New York City in a 30-month period under the liberalized state abortion law. The abortion culture is upon us. In one operating room, surgeons labor to save a 21-week-old baby; in the next, surgeons destroy, by abortion, another child, who can also be reckoned to be 21 weeks old. Where is the healing?

Plastic Bags

Look beyond the political arguments and see the fetus and what doctors do to it. An unborn baby's heartbeat begins between the eighteenth and twenty-fifth day; brain waves can be detected at seven weeks; at nine to ten weeks, the unborn squint, swallow and make a fist. Look at the marvelous photographs and see human life. Should these little human beings be killed unless it is to save the mother's life?

Other photos show this human life aborted, dropped onto surgical gauze or into plastic-bagged garbage pails. Take that human life by suction abortion and the body is torn apart, becoming a jumble of tiny arms and legs. In a D and C abortion, an instrument slices the body to pieces. Salt poisoning at nineteen weeks? The saline solution burns away the outer layer of the baby's skin. The ultimate is the hysterotomy (Caesarean section) abortion. As an operation, it can save mother and child; as an abortion it kills the child. Often, this baby fights for its life, breathes, moves and even cries. To see this, or the pictures of a plastic-bagged garbage can full of dead babies, well, it makes believers in right-to-life.

It's unfair to write this way, cry the super-abortionists, or to show the horrible photos. But Buchenwald and Dachau looked terrible, too. Abortions are always grisly tragedies. This truth must be restated at a time when medical administrators chatter about "cost-benefit analysis" factors in deciding who lives and who dies.

The "Good Death"

The utilitarian ethic is also common in the arguments of euthanasia advocates at work in six state legislatures. Their euphemisms drip like honey (should I say, cyanide?) just as they did in Germany—"death with dignity," the "good death." Their legal arguments fog the mind. Their mentality shakes me. One doctor, discussing the suicide-prone, wrote: "In such instances, positive euthanasia—a nice, smooth anesthetic to terminate life—appears preferable to suicide." Dr. Russell Sackett, author of the "Death With Dignity" bill in Florida, said: "Florida has 1,500 mentally retarded and mentally ill patients, 90 per cent of whom should be allowed to die." The German utilitarians had concluded the same when they led the first group of mental patients to the gas chamber at the Sonnestein Psychiatric Hospital in 1939. It bothers me that eugenicists in Germany organized the mass destruction of mental patients, and in the United States pro-abortionists now also serve in pro-euthanasia organizations. Sorry, but I see a pattern.

Utilitarianism isn't all abortion or euthanasia. Utilitarians ran the experiment in which syphilitic black men died through lack of penicillin. There are also experiments on free-clinic patients, students, the institutionalized. Senate hearings revealed that two experimental birth-control drugs were used on the "vulnerable" for purposes other than those approved by the Food and Drug Administration.

This monkeying around with people is relentless. Some medics would like to sterilize institutionalized people from here to breakfast. Psychosurgery is performed on hundreds of Americans annually, not to correct organic brain damage, but to alter their behavior. This chancy procedure, a first cousin of the now discredited prefrontal lobotomy that turned 50,000 Americans into human vegetables, is performed on unruly children and violence-prone prisoners.

Experimenters produce life outside the womb—combining sperm and ovum—and dispose of the human zygotes by pouring the solution down the sink drain. Recently scientists debated guidelines for experimenting with the live human fetus. To those considering the fetus as an organ, like, say, a kidney, Dr. Andre Hellegers of Georgetown University pointed out that fetuses have their own organs and cannot be considered organs themselves. How does one get consent from a live fetus? he asked. Or even from its donors—the parents who authorized the abortion?

Once fetal experimentation is sanctioned, are children to be next? Farfetched? No. In the *New England Journal of Medicine,* Dr. Franz Ingelfinger recently advocated removing the World Medical Association's absolute ban on experimenting with children and mental incompetents.

We can brake the tendencies of technocratic-minded doctors and administrators coldly concerned with "cost-benefit analysis." There was no such brake in Germany. After the first killings at Sonnestein, respected German doctors, not Nazi officials, killed 275,000 patients in the name of euthanasia. Many were curable. Eventually the doomed "undesirables" included epileptics, mental defectives, World War I amputees, children with "badly modeled ears" and "bed wetters."

Utilitarian Ethic

The worst barbarisms often have small beginnings. The logical extension of this utilitarian ethic was the mass exterminations in slave-labor camps. In "A Sign for Cain," Dr. Frederic Wertham tells how death-dealing technicians from German state hospitals (and their equipment) were moved to the camps in 1942 to begin the big job.

Could the "what is useful is good" mentality lead to such horror in the U.S.? Not so long as I am allowed to write like this—which German journalists couldn't. Not so long as right-to-life Americans can dispute—which Germans couldn't. The extremes of the utilitarian mentality rampaging today through medicine, the drug industry and government will be checked by our press, lawmakers and doctors, lawyers and clergymen holding to the traditional ethic. The Germans weren't blessed that way.

12

The Wife of Onan
and the Sons of Cain

John A. Miles, Jr.

Not long ago, I flew to Los Angeles for a major international conference on the study of religion, a *Mammutkongress* as a German report later described it, in which a dozen scholarly societies from around the world gathered to address the theme "Religion and the Humanization of Man." During the flight west I chanced to meet a fellow passenger who was a specialist in the neurophysiology of sexual attraction. He asked me about changes in the sexual morality of the churches and related matters. But I was brought up most sharply when he asked whether our conference would consider in any way the humanization of man by genetic modification. This indeed was not on the agenda, and the gravity of the omission taught me more than I learned in the conference itself.

An expert in comparative religion once observed that relations are usually quietest between religions that have least in common—like Christianity and Buddhism—and most acrimonious between religions that have most in common—like Christianity and Islam. Something similar obtains, it seems to me, in the relationship of religion to the humanities, on the one hand, and to natural science, on the other. Religion can quarrel with the humanities because they have a common language. But there is no common language for religion and natural science, and there is very little talk. It is as a result of this silence that religion so often finds itself struggling with a delayed impact of advances in natural science and the related technology.

More than the population explosion, more than the collapse of family life, it was the development of the contraceptive pill that precipitated the birth-control debate of the past decade. In a

From *National Review* (August 17, 1973), pp. 891-94. Reprinted by permission of *National Review*, 150 E. 35 Street, New York, N.Y. 10016.

similar way it has been the perfection of abortive techniques rather than a sudden outbreak of disrespect for life that has caused the present controversy over abortion. I do not mean to minimize socio-religious factors that are also at play. And yet if there is an aspect of the abortion debate that has been neglected, I think it must surely be the interplay between technology and values.

Can anyone doubt that as we now wrestle with the challenge posed by advances in embryology and antisepsis made a half-century and more ago, new challenges are brewing in other test tubes? In the present debate, for example, much has been made of the resemblance of the fetus to ourselves. It must be human because it looks so human. But what are we to make of *homo artificialis* as described by geneticist Bruce Wallace (*Saturday Review of Science,* February 1973)? *Homo artificialis,* the product of a quite conceivable genetic experiment, does not resemble man superficially. In an accompanying illustration, he lacks nose, mouth, ears, hair, and fingers. Nor is he capable of reproduction with man, though he can breed with other *hominibus artificialibus.* He is, however, capable of elaborate mental simulations, understands and attempts to follow the Golden Rule, and is capable of fear. Wallace says that taxonomically *homo artificialis* is not a member of the human species but adds, "Should I seek *human* company. . . I might choose the product of this genetic experimentation to many of my conspecific fellow men." If I ask, "Is the abortion of a *homo artificialis* a mortal sin?" and you feel that my question is out of place, then my point is made: In a technologically fertile society, the transformation of circumstance contributes as much as the erosion of basic morality to any conflicts that may bedevil us.

Our social commitment to technological transformation is of such long standing and such accumulated weight that only a secular apostasy of almost inconceivable violence could challenge it. However, in the absence of such an apostasy, it can still be instructive to consider the example of those small, recalcitrant communities that have managed, more or less, to resist the initial conversion. Certain American Pentecostals have been consistently opposed not only to abortion, birth control, and euthanasia but also to doctors, medication, life insurance, and banking. The well-known Amish community is opposed even to machinery and currency. Positions like theirs, however peculiar they seem on first acquaintance, do have an inner consistency. Either we are in the care of God, they argue, or we are not. If we are, do we not disparage His loving kindness and challenge His wisdom by the attempt to lengthen our days or enrich ourselves in bodily health or material possessions beyond what He chooses to provide? They guess, and shrewdly, that technology is a servant who takes over the house. In the Book of Genesis it is the descendants of Cain the murderer who invent metal-working, make musical instruments, and build towns. What the example of the Amish teaches about our present controversy is the inadequacy of saying, for example, that euthanasia follows abortion. Euthanasia does follow abortion, but it follows a great deal more than abortion, and the process of which abortion is part leads toward a great deal more than euthanasia.

The history of science and technology may be the story of the monster turning on Dr. Frankenstein, or it may be the story of Dr. Frankenstein taming the monster. It all depends on how you read it. Either way, however, it is instructive to step back a century or two and view life as it was lived before the introduction of a given technological blessing/curse. Since, in the present controversy, we are concerned with the technology of artificial birth control and medically safe abortion, we do well to ask how life was lived before these techniques were available.

Lost Foundlings

In a study entitled "Checks on Population Growth: 1750-1850" (*Scientific American*, February 1972), William L. Langer notes that the rate of marriage in the eighteenth century fluctuated according to economic conditions. Late marriage was the rule: Men married at 28 or 29, women at 25 or 26. However, there was a great deal of involuntary celibacy. Servants frequently did not marry. Women without income would live as dependents with relatives. Men joined the military.

In all of Germany except Prussia and in much of Switzerland, the procurement of the marriage license was far from a formality. Determined to eliminate pauperism, anxious to build a population of sturdy farmers and skilled artisans, a city like Württemberg could rule that "no one had the right to produce children whom he was unable to support and who thereby became the responsibility of the population." Thus in 1830, there was only one marriage among 121 inhabitants of Württemberg, and only one among 236 in 1854.

England did not ration marriage licenses in this way. Rather, after the humane fashion of the English, the New Poor Law of 1834 merely required that paupers live in designated poorhouses and that males and females be separately housed, even if they were married.

The most important check on population growth, however, was not enforced celibacy but infanticide. Even as late as 1878, 6 percent of all deaths in England were the result of infanticide. Note that the statistic does not report that 6 percent of infant deaths were by killing but that 6 percent of all deaths in the population were the deaths of murdered infants. To put that statistic in perspective, consider that deaths by automobile accident account for only 3 percent of the total deaths per annum in the United States.

Infanticide was against the law, of course. Penalties for it ranged up to death by drowning and burial alive; but they had little effect. Infants were dispatched by starvation and strangulation. They were poisoned with gin. Their skulls were broken with hairbrushes. They were exposed in church doorways or on the streets. And, perhaps most commonly, they were "overlaid"; that is, smothered as they slept in bed with their mothers. Edwin Lankester, a journalist of the day, reports that he never knew of a woman punished for killing her own offspring, no matter how flagrant the circumstances.

Voices were raised against infanticide, of course, and social remedies were applied. But as is so often the case when an attempted remedy is purely social, they only compounded the problem. One Thomas Coran, a retired admiral, organized a foundling hospital in London in 1741 and in 1756 was granted government funds for it. A bell was hung outside the front gate of the hospital so that abandoning parents needed only ring it and run. And ring it they did. Coran's hospital was inundated. During the four years from 1756 to 1760, fifteen thousand foundlings were accepted. Unfortunately, 10,600 of these died; in 1760 the hospital had to curtail its activities.

Other foundling hospitals grew up around the country, but it would be overkind to describe these as charitable institutions. Jonas Hardway, another contemporary observer, called them "these slaughterhouses of infants." Popularly, they were known as "baby farms" and those who staffed them as "killing nurses" and "she-butchers." In the "baby farms," infants were commonly dispatched with a concoction known as "Godfrey's treacle," a blend of opium, treacle, and sassafras. Ten gallons or twelve thousand doses of "Godfrey's treacle" were sold in Coventry each week. When Richard Carlile, an early advocate of birth control, said, "it is a question if infanticide ever prevailed in any country more than in our own," his statement went unchallenged, though Langer's modern study suggests that conditions were perhaps worse in France. In 1863 the *Morning Star* wrote that infanticide "is positively becoming a national institution."

If infanticide is not equally widespread in our own day, the credit surely must go to the technology of birth control. And so if the technological management of human existence from hospital cradle to hospital grave is a prospect dismal to contemplate, we may take some grim comfort that the alternatives are hardly less humane.

Another technologically generated conflict, directly involved in the abortion debate, concerns the rise of Women's Liberation. Am I in favor of Women's Liberation? I have asked myself. Of course, I answered at first. Then I said simply, yes. Then, not very. Now I say, I don't know. For it is plain, on a moment's reflection, that the liberation in question is primarily technological liberation from pregnancy and from the web of social roles deriving therefrom, and who can foresee clearly enough where that web will prove to have supported us and where restrained to declare so soon either his support or his opposition? Consider:

> The one thing wrong with my many mental pictures of Sally and our child was that I wasn't in any of them. All I could picture was Sally and the baby, and the reason was that Sally made it perfectly obvious to me that that was how she pictured it. I don't think she used the pronoun "we" at all, after she knew that she was pregnant. For her our marriage seemed to have ended on that day. From then on she said "I'll," never "we'll.". . . It took me months to articulate it to myself, but my one function in Sally's life had been to get her pregnant. I had performed it, and that was that. All she had needed of me was my seed. I gave it and that was that. In all other respects she was self-sufficient. She didn't even say thank you for the seed.

I don't know what that quotation, from Larry McMurtry's *All My Friends Are Going To Be Strangers,* suggests to you, but to me it suggests that if abortion is the concern only of the woman and her physician, then psychologically if not logically, so is motherhood. In other words, the day is past when "unwed mother" automatically meant "deserted mother." A friend of mine is considering having a child by a man she knows she would never marry. Those who could still say of her pregnancy, "Some guy got her in trouble," do not appreciate the impact of technology on morals.

Or consider this, from Walker Percy's *Love in the Ruins:*

> "It's not your fault. People grow away from each other. Spiritual growth is the law of life. Our obligation is to be true to ourselves and to relate to this law of life."
> "Isn't marriage a relation?"
> "Our marriage is a collapsed morality, like a burnt-out star which collapses into itself, gives no light and is heavy heavy heavy."

Merde. Spiritual growth, thus individually understood, may be a commitment, but it is not the law of life. You may sacrifice everything and everyone to it if you wish, but (forgive my impertinence) you will not die if you do not. As Philip Rieff has so searingly demonstrated, unconditional commitment to one's own spiritual growth is the solvent which dissolves absolutely every relationship, leaving a world in which one is not only, in Kafka's phrase, "a sect unto himself," but also a family unto himself. I find more than a trace of that corrosive in Justice Blackmun's opinion inasmuch as he chose to base it on the individual woman's right to privacy. For my own part, however, I do not so much question the woman's right to privacy as wonder about the implications of her desire for it, and of my own.

Nena and George O'Neill write in the preface of their best-selling *Open Marriage:*

> Two consistent threads ran through all our interviews: One was the desire for freedom, and the other a longing for relatedness to another—a search for a deeply personal and mutual commitment in a relationship that would not bind or constrict growth.

I do not believe, in the abstract, that those two threads are consistent with each other, but rather that they are finally contradictory. And yet they will not fight to a standstill, for one of them, the thread of freedom, has behind it the weight of a major, technologically generated trend; viz., the American trend to do alone and unaided much that in an earlier era we did in consort.

Self-service shopping eliminates the need to talk to the grocer. Air-conditioning permits one to stay indoors on hot nights. Campers eliminate the social complication of the hotel, and cheap yachts the interpersonal ordeal of the ocean cruise. I count myself no Luddite; and particularly for the class (my own) which used to perform the named services, the gifts of technology are balm in Gilead. More mixed a blessing, however, is a spreading confidence in the total adequacy of the individual, a triumph of privacy that, in works like *Open Marriage*, captures even the bedroom.

The triumph of privacy might be innocuous enough if each could be not only a sect and a family unto himself but a nation as well. Alas, it would seem that this is not to be. Totalitarianism is by definition the elimination of every independent organizational unit that might stand between the individual and the organized total state. Some of the proponents of abortion reform seem to regard the Supreme Court decision as their liberation from tyrannization by the Roman Catholic Church with its infallible pope. But as Gordon Zahn has pointed out, they naively expect that once the Court has spoken, the matter should be settled for Catholic consciences as well as for their own. Catholics stand as heretics before a secular infallibility, repeating with a new referent Galileo's *"Eppur si muove."* And if the heresy dies out, as well it may, there will die with it some of the power the Catholic Church might use to interpose a larger protective unit between the privatized citizen and his government. Whatever the truth of the abortion cause, I find that prospect sobering.

Unfound Foundlings

What will be the machinery of abortion enforcement? None, one might think at first: No one is ever required to have an abortion, and moreover this is a judicial decision not an act of legislation. But of course the laws are being rewritten, and I beg leave to doubt that they will always respect the conscience of, say, a physician in a remote area.

In any area of public policy, legality, encouragement, and

coercion constitute a continuum. According to the *Chicago Daily News* (March 26, 1973), State Representative Webber Borchers (R.) has introduced a bill into the Illinois House that would require the state to provide free and voluntary vasectomies and tubal ligations to persons who have cohabited in Illinois for a year and have a combined income of less than $5,000 a year. If the couple's combined income is less than $3,000 a year, each could get a free vasectomy or tubal ligation—plus a $100 check from the state. The program would cost the state $2 million. Now sterilization has always been a legal operation. Rep. Borchers simply wants to provide a $100 incentive for it. But now that abortion is also legal, nothing would prevent him or some other legislator from providing an incentive for abortion—a bounty on the fetus, as it were.

Neither of these measures, of course, mentions race. Borchers' only (perverse) requirement for sterilization is cohabitation. The services in question would be available to blacks and whites alike. And yet if I were a black man earning $100,000 a year, I would still react to these proposals as to a newspaper advertisement for a brick bungalow in a desirable location. It does not surprise me that Jean Noble, Executive Director of the National Council of Negro Women, believes that "abortion is genocidal, a method of limiting the black population." It does not surprise me, in other words, to find a distant-early-warning alarm in black people to any public policy in which the word "unwanted" is allowed so prominent a role. Whites who may find such imagined threats to black life remote do well to recall Goering's response to the complaint that too many gentiles were going to the concentration camps. He said, "I decide who is a Jew."

Money, of course, is one of the crasser incentives. In Kurt Vonnegut's "Welcome to the Monkey House," men are persuaded more insidiously to make society's goals their own. In Vonnegut's fantasy, sexual gratification is not available outside "Ethical Suicide Parlors," manned by virgin hostesses in purple body stockings, prepared for their work with degrees in psychology and nursing. Because of automation, most men are unemployed and spend their time watching television and hearing, every 15 minutes, a public-service announcement urging them to "pay a call to the nearest Ethical Suicide Parlor and find out how friendly and understanding a Hostess [can] be." We may be far from Vonnegut's fantasy world, and yet I confess I was reminded of his hostesses as I read the following published description of counselors in a New York abortion clinic:

> A counselor may be a nurse, a social worker, a psychologist, or, in many cases, an unspecialized college graduate who is bright, friendly, calm, empathetic, believes strongly in the right to abortion, probably has had one herself, and is present as surrogate friend. The best counselors work hard and successfully to allay the patient's worst fears, listen to and help with all sorts of problems, and stand by her while the doctor is at work, holding her hand, stroking her forehead, *talking all the while to take her mind off the moment.* [Emphasis added.]

One wonders, given the current enlightened (à la Kubler-Ross) management of death, what the liberal reaction would be to a nurse who talked all the while to take the dying patient's mind off the moment. But I digress.

Is Life Fundamental?

National Review (June 22) reports Senator James Buckley's speech on behalf of the Human Life Amendment to the Constitution. Senator Buckley is reported to be reluctant to take the route of constitutional amendment: "My decision was not lightly taken, for I believe that only matters of permanent and fundamental interest are properly the subject for constitutional amendment." Though I would not support the amendment as framed, I personally welcome the prospect of a constitutional debate, for—unlike Senator Buckley—I am convinced that an issue of permanent and fundamental interest is indeed joined. The issue is not abortion but rather our national response to the coming technology of social science.

Even if that response is to be an unqualified and systematic negative (hardly to be presumed in advance of the debate), it would be well to take the time to utter it. The much maligned B. F. Skinner has faced an essential implication not just of behavioral psychology but of social science as such; namely, that if social science is indeed science, then it can and will generate technology and even industry. What the counter-utopian literature from Orwell and Huxley down to Vonnegut and Burgess suggests is that this most recent technology is a sin. And maybe it is. But a future generation might regard our horror of social innoculation with the same puzzlement with which we regard the Jehovah's Witnesses' horror of blood transfusion. Either way we are party to a debate that the framers of the Constitution could scarcely have foreseen on an issue as broad as the construction of society itself. If we find the Foundling Fathers by implication opposed to the new technology, then let us draw the implication in so many words.

Failing to do that, we may expect that this technology—like earlier technology—will be exploited in a privatized, random fashion and will surprise us at some future date with an ugly public quarrel. In Arthur Koestler's most recent novel, a dozen scientists meet in Switzerland to discuss the survival of the human species and to consider the advisability of drafting a letter to the President like Einstein's famous letter to Roosevelt. A neurophysiologist rises with a novel proposal:

> It is quite simple, my dear colleagues. You collect a thousand volunteers. You pay them. You do not tell them what the experiment is about. You tell them the pills are for having nice dreams while you sleep. During the treatments you arrange for various incidents to occur. The office boss is unpleasant to the subject. He is pushed in the subway by an *agent provocateur.* His wife starts flirting with his best friend. . . . If the subjects pass all these tests with stoic fortitude, the product can be put on the market. When its effects are shown on television, the use of the product will spread very quickly. It will also spread across the Iron Curtain and the Chinese Wall. Then the tampering. . . can be done with public approval. Otherwise it will have to be done anyway.

The neurophysiologist's proposal is greeted with horror. He himself is a bit ostracized at the final session. That night he reflects in his room that he

> did not feel justified in telling them that the experiment was actually on its way. Soon after his return the team would have received and tabulated the first results. Then we shall see. . . .

This is the sort of surprise I should like to see the United States avoid. It may, of course, be unavoidable. However, if the coming constitutional debate can somehow correct its course to approach abortion as a subheading under dangers of social technology rather than simply as a subheading under murder, then there is hope.

13

Equal Protection

Richard Landau

At the conclusion of a high-school ice hockey game at the Boston Garden last March, highspirited fans tossed a few tons of debris into the air and onto the ice. A few days later, newspapers reported that amid the crumpled paper bags, greasy napkins, programs and hot dog wrappers, custodians had found a dead fetus.

It would be idle to speculate on how it came to be there. But the fact that it was there should come as no surprise at a time of extraordinary public and private ambiguity as to the moral and legal status of the unborn child.

Massachusetts, like many other states, is embroiled annually in a legislative debate as to whether or not its abortion law should be "reformed." The law permits abortion, but only if necessary to preserve the physical or mental health of the mother. Amid the *Sturm und Drang*, neither side has paid attention to a little-publicized decision of the Massachusetts Supreme Judicial Court that has direct bearing—philosophically if not legally—on some of the issues central to the abortion controversy. The case in question was a civil matter, but the arguments raised bring into sharp focus the basic question: Does a viable fetus have rights under law that are independent of its mother's?

The facts in the case are not exceptional. In 1969, a pregnant woman was being attended by a physician who had been her obstetrician for two previous successful pregnancies. As her third pregnancy was nearing term, she noticed that fetal movement had stopped, which she reported to her physician's partner who was on duty on the day of her visit. He suggested that certain tests be made in a local hospital, but these apparently did not clearly

From *National Review* (January 19, 1973), pp. 87, 107. Reprinted by permission of *National Review*, 150 E. 35 Street, New York, N.Y. 10016.

establish whether the fetus was still alive. Not long afterward, the fetus was stillborn.

According to the mother, the physicians had not advised her that she had Rh-negative blood, and, she alleged, they had not taken proper steps to make possible the survival of the baby. The parents, as administrators of the estate of the stillborn infant girl, sued the physicians under the Massachusetts Wrongful Death Statute.

Although common law makes ample provision for recovery of damages for wrongful injury, there is no provision for damages in the case of wrongful death. In most jurisdictions, including Massachusetts, a statute makes up for this gap in common law. In some states, recovery is based on the pecuniary loss suffered by the survivors. Thus, the survivors of a stockbroker could expect to collect more than the survivors of an itinerant handyman, all other things being equal. In Massachusetts and in several other states, however, the statute awards damages on the basis of culpability and is, therefore, essentially punitive.

The parents filed their action under the Wrongful Death Statute in Middlesex County Superior Court. In so doing, they (and their attorneys) were knowingly raising a direct challenge to previous Massachusetts court decisions in cases of this kind. For, in all previous rulings in the Commonwealth, the courts had held that a fetus that is not born alive is not a "person" and its survivors cannot recover damages under the Wrongful Death Statute.

Attorneys for the physicians filed a demurrer to the complaint pointing to those prior decisions and arguing that there was no cause of action: The fetus was not a person. The lower court sustained the demurrer and subsequently the Supreme Judicial Court, the Commonwealth's highest tribunal, affirmed the decision of the lower court. Unless the issue is carried into the federal system, then, the status of the fetus under civil law in Massachusetts remains what it was. That is, the fetus is a nonperson.

Although the courts did no more than affirm the status quo, the arguments raised in the briefs touch upon some fascinating issues, not only for Massachusetts, and not only for civil law. And the decision of the higher court, when examined in the context of the briefs, raises more questions than it answers.

The defense brief offered a wide range of arguments as to why the court should refuse to hear the case, each of which was disputed by the plaintiffs. Two of the arguments had a direct bearing on the abortion issue. They are closely related to one another:

1. It is difficult and at times impossible to determine pre-trauma viability of the fetus *in utero.* As a result, the only rule that can be applied without uncertainty is one based exclusively on whether or not there was a live birth.

2. The fetus is not a person prior to birth because it is a part of the mother, and because the commonly understood meaning of the word fetus does not include person, and the legal usage of person does not include fetus.

The court in this case accepted the first argument in its entirety, and, regarding the second, indicated that if the word person is to be applied to a fetus, that determination would have to be made by the legislature and not the courts.

Regarding the first argument, attorneys for the plaintiffs argued that medicine has made great strides in recent decades, and that viability is no longer as difficult to determine as it once was. Furthermore, they pointed out, holding to *live birth* rather than *viability* as the sole deciding factor in whether a case is actionable could result in anomalies and absurdities. For example, they raised a question posed hypothetically in an earlier Ohio case: Supposing that twins suffered the same prenatal injury, and one died before birth and the other shortly after. Should there be a cause of action for one and not the other?

One could carry the illustrations further. If the unborn children of two women suffered injury as a result of negligence or willful action by another, the fetus that suffered the more serious trauma and that as a result died in the womb would have no rights under law, but the one whose injury was the lesser and who was born alive, dying a few hours later, would have an estate.

The issue is complicated by the fact that "birth" itself is not a precisely defined moment in time. How would the court cope with a case involving a fetus that was alive on leaving the birth canal but which died before the umbilical cord was cut? Was it "born"? Was it ever a "person"? At precisely what point does a fetus become a person? When it crowns? When it cries?

At no point in its decision did the court come to grips with the core of the difficulty: Conception, fetal development, birth, life and death are not distinct historic episodes, but are instead vaguely defined and overlapping segments of a continuum. At some point a fetus is not viable, and at some point it is: At some point it is unborn, and at some point it is born. The moments of transition are murky. Life tends to be untidy.

The court, however, accepted the defense argument. But the judge's preference for what he called an "easily administered rule" is surely not compelling; if we were governed in every aspect of our civil lives by that principle, we could dispense with lawyers and judges.

The second argument—over what is a person—comes even closer to confronting the abortion issue. The question of whether or not the word person includes fetus can be argued semantically, but that path is not very fruitful. The plaintiffs chose another course, a course that may possibly have implications for the abortion controversy.

In their brief, the plaintiffs referred to a dissenting opinion filed in a recent and similar case in Michigan. One of the appellate judges there pointed out that the state and federal courts have for years struggled with the meaning of the word person as it is used in the Bill of Rights. Did the word, for example, apply to a convict? an alien? an Indian? a black? The rights of each of these to be considered a person has at one time or another been challenged, and in every case the courts have turned aside the challenge and applied the word, and the rights, to the person. The Michigan judge then pointed out that even corporate entities are considered persons entitled to the protection of the Fourteenth Amendment. If an inanimate entity like a corporation or a labor union can be a legal person and therefore guaranteed equal protection under the law, why not a fetus, he asked. The dissenting Michigan judge then cited a Supreme Court decision to show that the Fourteenth Amendment applied to children as well as to adults, and wondered why an unborn child who is no less human than one already born should be denied equal protection of the law. He concluded:

> To say that one may kill some human beings—those who have been born—and be held responsible under the law, and that one may kill other human beings—those who have not been born—and go free, is a denial of equal protection of the laws and ought not to be condoned by any court.

The Massachusetts Supreme Judicial Court chose to ignore the "equal protection" argument. Some day, however, if a case of this sort should find its way to the United States Supreme Court on the question of the applicability of the Fourteenth Amendment to unborn children, the decision might be fraught with meaning for the abortion controversy. Theoretically, of course, it would be possible to apply the word person to fully formed and viable fetuses, while denying the status implicit in that word to the not-yet-viable fetus or the embryo that precedes it. But what would we then say of trauma suffered by an embryo who lives long enough to become a person and then dies? Had *he* no right to life?

And, if he did, what then shall we make of abortion "reform"?

Part III

Compulsory Sterilization: Population Control or Genocide?

During the last decade an increasing number of people have looked upon sterilization as an acceptable means of fertility control. Yet those who have been sterilized against their will, or without adequate knowledge of the operation, are not so complacent. It seems that one person's solution to the overcrowded welfare rolls is another's genocide. The use of government funds to sterilize children and mentally incompetent people has been ended by Federal District Court Judge Gerhard Gesell's March 1974 decision. Gesell ruled that these people did not have enough knowledge or the judgment to meet the standard of informed consent. He also commented that the threat to withdraw welfare funds was no way to induce "voluntary consent." The article by Jack Slater illustrates the dilemmas that led to the court's decision.

The essay by Jan Charles Gray surveys the legal background of a possible sterilization law. Indeed, he finds compulsory sterilization after two or three children would have a legal basis. Anne and Paul Ehrlich also espouse sterilization as a means of fertility control, and they hope that education will lead people to voluntary sterilization. Garrett Hardin, on the other hand, despairs of anything but coercion to limit the number of people on earth.

14

Sterilization:
Newest Threat to the Poor

Jack Slater

This is a story about a crime and a special kind of death in the land of equal opportunity. Last June, on a warm, unsuspecting morning in Montgomery, Ala., two young black girls were wheeled into a hospital operating room and rendered sexually sterile by tubal ligation because, somewhere in their neighborhood, somewhere on their block, so the authorities said, "boys were hanging around." Later it was learned that the girls and their parents were on welfare and that their welfare status had some direct connection with the sterilizations.

Four months have passed since that June morning, yet it is still difficult to comprehend fully the enormity of what actually happened to those young girls—difficult to digest the news of other sterilization cases reported in the nation, or the latest revelations that since 1964 more than one thousand American women, most of them black and all of them poor, have been forced to submit to involuntary sterilization. It is difficult even to understand what such a crime supposes itself to be saying, what it presumes itself to be wanting, what circumstances would permit it or what it portends.

Here are a few details:

— On June 13, two representatives of the federally financed Montgomery Community Action Agency called on Mrs. Minnie Relf, an illiterate welfare mother of four, to tell her that her two youngest daughters, Mary Alice, fourteen, and Minnie Lee, twelve, needed some shots. (Agency officials, incidentally, have claimed that young Minnie Lee Relf is mentally retarded.) The nature of the shots, according to Mrs. Relf, seemed to be uncertain; but, believing that the agency had the best interest of her daughters'

From *Ebony* Magazine 28 (October 1973), pp. 150-56. Copyright 1973 by Johnson Publishing Co., Inc. Reprinted by permission.

health in mind, Mrs. Relf consented—and subsequently signed an informed consent release. "I put an X on a paper," she said later. And, armed with that "X", the agency, which operates a family planning clinic also federally supported, affected its own version of population control—ostensibly because of those "boys. . . hanging around." (After the Relf case came to light, it was discovered that for the past fifteen months, federally sponsored birth control clinics around the nation have sterilized at least eighty other minors.)

— In July, at a crowded press conference in New York City, Nial Ruth Cox, an angry, unwed black mother, accompanied by her lawyer from the American Civil Liberties Union (ACLU), revealed that eight years earlier, when she was pregnant with her only child, she too had been forced to undergo permanent sterilization in New Bern, N. C. Miss Cox, who is twenty-six years old, had agreed to the sterilization, she said, because she had been told it would be a temporary measure and also because she had been warned that if she did not agree, her family would cease to receive welfare payments. After a New York doctor recently told her she could never have another child, Miss Cox, an alert intelligent woman by almost anyone's standards, learned that the physician who rendered her sterile had justified the operation by declaring her to be "mentally deficient." Referring to the operation during an interview, Miss Cox told *Ebony:* "I feel like half a woman. No man wants half a woman. A man is going to look for someone who can give him a child. I don't even look anymore."

— A few days following that press conference, Mrs. Carol Brown, a thirty-year-old, pregnant mother of four near Aiken, S. C., became publicly outraged at her own hapless situation. On the welfare rolls since February when her husband began serving a prison term for grand larceny, Mrs. Brown, who is white, was due to have her fifth baby soon. Contacting the three physicians in town, she was told that none of them could deliver her child unless she first agreed to be sterilized. It seemed that Mrs. Brown, as a welfare mother of more than three children, had more babies than any of the doctors could conscionably allow the overburdened state taxpayers to support.

After the details of those three cases were revealed, news of other sterilizations were disclosed in the same states as well as in Texas, Florida and California. Twenty-six states currently have eugenic sterilization statutes, but the state which appears to be the most thorough and most determined in its pursuit of sterilization is North Carolina.

Since 1933, the state of North Carolina, through its Eugenics Commission, has ordered "thousands" of sterilizations in the name of "the public good," says Mrs. June Stallings, executive secretary of the commission. During the past nine years, 1,107 sterilizations were ordered by the commission. In 1972, 70 such operations were approved from 116 petitions presented to the commission. Since the first of this year, 13 sterilizations were approved from 32 petitions.

Although the Eugenics Commission has declined to reveal the racial breakdowns of the number of sterilizations authorized since 1964, Brenda Feigen Fasteau, the ACLU attorney who represents Nial Ruth Cox, says: "As far as I can determine, the statistics reveal that since 1964 approximately 65 percent of the women sterilized in North Carolina were black and approximately 35 percent were white."

But one doesn't need to know too much about involuntary sterilization in North Carolina to detect that racism is involved—and beyond mere racism, some unspeakable wish to control black population growth by force. ("I think it has finally penetrated the white mind that people of color outnumber the white people of the world," declares Bruce Hilton, a noted medical ethics specialist and director of the National Center for Bio-Ethics.) In fact, to detect the racism, one doesn't need to know too much about forced sterilizations in the other states. In Alabama, for example, more than 50 percent of the involuntary sterilizations authorized this past year by the State Health Department were performed on black people. And in Aiken, S. C., black women were subjects of sixteen of the eighteen sterilizations paid for by Medicaid and performed by a Dr. Clovis H. Pierce, a white, forty-year-old former Army physician. (Incidentally, medical payments to Dr. Pierce have totaled $60,000 in the past eighteen months, according to Aiken County Hospital records.)

In *Law and Society Review* (August 1968), Julius Paul, of the Walter Reed Army Institute of Research, cited the growing use of punitive sterilization measures. He wrote:

> "Numerous [state] legislative attempts have included sterilization as part of a program of recommended punitive action that may include the loss of welfare benefits, the imprisonment and/or fining of the mother, the loss of custody of the children, and various combinations of the

above. The arguments in favor of these proposals are couched in economic terms (the rising costs of welfare services), or "moral" terms (the alarming rise in the rate of illegitimacy, especially among Negroes), and sometimes covertly or overtly on racial grounds.

Racism, however, isn't the only passion surrounding the sterilization scandal. In addition to color—and apparently greed, other national themes compound the issue. As Julius Paul suggests, hatred of the poor—black and white—is certainly a leitmotiv. ("At least fourteen states have considered or are considering legislation designed to coerce women receiving welfare to submit to sterilization," says Susan LaMont, a spokeswoman for the Women's National Abortion Action Coalition.) Moreover, as others have suggested, sexism, or hatred of women, may also be involved. ("Have you come across any women sterilizing other women involuntarily?" asks Bruce Hilton.)

"The sterilization issue affects all of us," declares feminist Gloria Steinem, "but especially women, and especially minority women. The government thinks it not only has the right to tap our phones but to interfere in all areas of our personal lives, including governing our very bodies."

Yet the sterilization scandal seems to expose something more elemental and more subterranean than hatred of women, or even hatred of unwed mothers. For, at some subconscious level concealed beneath a plethora of fabricated justifications about family planning and welfare cheating, hatred of sex may also be involved.

"I don't think we can ignore the puritan overtones surrounding forced sterilization," says Bruce Hilton. " 'Sex is bad'—or so the puritan will tell you. And when you are a puritan, you can justify stepping into another person's life and forcing him to do what you think is right, because he, after all, is sinning." Furthermore: "The whole paternalism thing in the South might also be involved. I think it is true that otherwise decent, God-fearing, church-going people still feel that God has given them the black man as a responsibility. And that kind of paternalism says that if this woman isn't smart enough to stop having children, then it is my responsibility to help her. After all," he adds, "the most horrendous crimes are done in the name of doing good for somebody else."

But what set of precedents or circumstances could have allowed such a crime to take place?

Dr. Arlene P. Bennett suggests that American genetics dogma is itself the precedent. Not long ago, shortly after the hysteria about genetic screening for sickle cell anemia swept across the country, Dr. Bennett, a public school physician in Elizabeth, N. J., became alarmed at the implications involved in such screening. Suspecting that the hysteria was creating a climate in which sterilizations for sickle cell would become acceptable, she set about to do a little research into the history of eugenic sterilizations in America.

"As early as 1897," Dr. Bennett writes in an unpublished article, "a Dr. F. Hoyt Pilcher castrated forty-four boys and fourteen girls at a Kansas Institution for the Feebleminded. . . . In 1907, a Dr. Harry C. Sharpe boasted of having vasectomized between six hundred and seven hundren boys at an Indiana reformatory. . . . [Elsewhere in America] the candidates for sterilization included the mentally ill, mentally retarded, epileptics, those infected with TB or VD, prostitutes, criminals and paupers—all conditions believed to be inherited at the time."

In an interview, Dr. Bennett will tell you: "I also discovered that in the early part of the century, sterilizations were used against 'undesirable' Southern European immigrants. Primarily because of their so-called 'innate inferiority,' their poverty and illiteracy. Does that sound familiar?" she asks with a chuckle. Then referring again to sickle cell anemia and the current sterilization issue, she adds: "Any phenomenon in our history of popularized or politicized genetic dogma has ultimately led to thoughts about abortions, therapeutic abortions and sterilizations."

Thus, the climate which permitted America's first recorded, mass castration of the "genetically unfit" in 1897 led, link by link, to the sterilization of two Alabama black girls in 1973.

Since the disclosure of the Alabama case (and the North and South Carolina cases), nothing much has changed, however. Senator Edward Kennedy has held a Senate subcommittee hearing on the issue. Six federal and state investigations are now being conducted, including two by the U.S. Justice Department and the Office of Economic Opportunity. And new federal guidelines forbidding sterilization without informed consent have been issued by the Department of Health, Education and Welfare. Yet for all of the official sound and fury, involuntary sterilizations will probably continue, since the subcommittee hearings and the present investigations are merely fact-finding efforts, and the new

Table 1. STATE AUTHORIZING STERILIZATION
(AS OF FEBRUARY 1971)

State	Mentally Ill or Mentally Defective	Criminals (Certain Categories)	Epileptics
Alabama	x		
Arizona	x		x
California	x	x	
Connecticut*	x	x	
Delaware	x	x	x
Georgia	x	x	
Idaho	x	x	x
Indiana	x		x
Iowa	x	x	
Maine	x		
Michigan	x	x	
Minnesota*	x		
Mississippi	x		x
Montana			x
Nebraska			x
New Hampshire	x		x
North Carolina	x	x	x
Oklahoma	x	x	x
Oregon	x	x	x
South Carolina	x		x
South Dakota	x		
Utah	x	x	x
Vermont*	x		
Virginia	x		x
West Virginia	x		x
Wisconsin	x	x	

*The sterilization statutes of these states are voluntary in nature. All of the other states have compulsory sterilization laws.

guidelines are, as an HEW spokesman confesses, impotent direc-
tives without any "police" powers. "Until we adequately police
them," says Dr. Carl Shultz, director of HEW's office of
population affairs, "the guidelines aren't going to be fully
effective." Which is, it seems, the United States Government's
way of saying that the poor and all of those people luckless
enough to have been labeled "mentally defective" still have no

rights which any physician need respect.

At the moment, the only recourse seems to be a lawsuit. On behalf of Nial Ruth Cox, the ACLU is suing the North Carolina Eugenics Commission and others for $1 million in damages. And through the Southern Poverty Law Center, the Relf family in Alabama has filed a suit against OEO and HEW for $5 million in damages—a suit which, in addition to the sterilization claims, seeks damages for the clinic's use of an experimental, federally uncertified birth control drug, Depo-provera, on the Relf's oldest daughter, Katy, seventeen.

In the meantime, most observers have overlooked a tragic irony to the entire issue of involuntary sterilization. For if control of black population growth is one of the ruling motives behind such sterilization, it should be noted that in recent years birth rates even among poor women "have—*voluntarily*—dropped far greater than rates among the affluent," says John Robbins, director of the Planned Parenthood Federation of America. In the 1966-70 period birth rates for women from poor families, he says, declined by 21 percent, compared to the drop of 18 percent among women in the middle class.

Meanwhile, the scandal itself continues—and continues to evoke a kind of paralyzed outrage from black people. Black U.S. congressmen have written angry letters to HEW Secretary Caspar Weinberger. NAACP and Urban League officials have made speeches full of heat and black newspapers have been justifiably indignant. But to date no united effort on the part of blacks—and no local, state or national movement composed of blacks—to stop the threat has been initiated.

Apparently only one white woman, Gloria Steinem, has publicly sounded the battle cry by urging that forced sterilization "be fought and fought as a coalition issue."

"I don't think," says Dr. Arlene Bennett, "that black people, black doctors or black leaders can sit by any longer. We must stop individual professionals from playing God."

It is quite clear that there is already an army of black women whose names are Nial Ruth Cox. And the contempt which has embraced them may—unless we prevent it—soon encircle more of us, even as it will always encircle Mary Alice and Minnie Lee Relf. Somehow, soon, in some unmistakable, uncompromising way, we must say that we have had enough.

15

Compulsory Sterilization in a Free Society: Choices and Dilemmas

Jan Charles Gray

The problem of surplus population has traditionally been associated with the undeveloped nations of the world. Yet recently we have become aware that overpopulation also presents a pressing dilemma for the industrialized world. Despite optimistic news reports, the population problem has not been mooted by a decline in the birthrate. The headlines often emphasize this decline but fail to alert us that the growth rate has not fallen. Since the postwar "baby boom" women are now of child-bearing age, and although the birthrate may be low for a few years, the overall capacity of these women to produce children remains the same. This means that in years to come an increase in the birthrate and a concomitant substantial increase in the growth rate could be triggered.

Congress has responded by forming a Presidential Commission on Population Growth to conduct a probing inquiry into various aspects of the problem. The Commission's major finding was that population growth in the United States must be stabilized before the nation can begin to solve its other domestic social problems. Not surprisingly, the Commission Report focused on the "unwanted birth." While rejecting compulsory measures, it proposed the liberalization of abortion laws, and recommended that federal, state, and local governments make funds available to support abortion services in states with liberalized statutes. Additionally, it was thought that abortion should be specifically included in comprehensive health insurance benefits, both public and private.

In light of this increasing concern with population growth, many proposed solutions will be advocated in years to come. This article examines one statutory answer to the population problem, a compulsory sterilization statute (the Population Control Statute) which would require the sterilization of a spouse after the birth of two children. At present, this may seem a drastic measure, neither socially desirable nor politically feasible, but prevailing social and political attitudes could quickly and dramatically be transformed under the press of overpopulation. But even if one acknowledges that a compulsory sterilization statute would have little immediate legislative success, the discussion and consideration of it as an alternative might suggest other, less onerous governmental or private methods for controlling population growth. Indeed, stimulating thought concerning what can be done today to avert future compulsory measures is itself a reason to discuss compulsory sterilization.

Compulsory Sterilization: A Constitutional Analysis

Any enactment of legislation restricting the right of individuals to determine the number of children that may be born to them would raise serious constitutional issues. In this regard a Population Control Statute could be challenged on many grounds by diverse interest groups. Catholics might contend that the enactment was a violation of their first amendment right to the free exercise of religion. Blacks, as well as other minorities, might charge that the statute was an attempt at "genocide" and therefore a violation of the Fourteenth Amendment's equal protection clause. Finally, a universal concern would be that compulsory sterilization constituted not only an invasion of the body and a denial of the right of procreation, but also an interference with the right of marital privacy. The Fifth and Fourteenth Amendments' guarantee of "due process" would be the basis for the contention that the statute's reach would deprive an individual of basic civil liberties and hence be unconstitutional.

This article, however, proposes that sufficient precedent exists to sustain a Population Control Statute and examines the popular notion that compulsory population control is not possible in the United States. In support of the proposed Population Control Statute, analysis of present case law and a probing inquiry into the present and future goals of our society may reveal that the precedential value of certain cases is greater than formerly believed. The solace some have taken from Supreme Court pronouncements regarding procreation and the right to marital privacy may be unfounded and reliance on those cases overstated.

1. Due Process Considerations

Although not specifically guaranteed by the Constitution, certain fundamental rights and protected interests are considered basic and therefore protected under the due process clause of the Fourteenth Amendment. This expanding notion of fundamental rights, though a current one, seems to be implanted firmly in constitutional doctrine. Included in the growing list of protected interests one finds: procreation, marriage, marital privacy, fairness in the criminal process, education, interstate travel, and voting. The focus of concern with a Population Control Statute would be a precise delineation of the scope of two fundamental interests, procreation and marital privacy.

Some may believe that two landmark Supreme Court decisions, *Skinner v. Oklahoma,* 316 U.S. 535 (1942) and *Griswold v. Connecticut,* 381 U.S. 479 (1965), may foreclose debate on the possible constitutionality of a statute regulating procreation in marriage. The Supreme Court in *Skinner* treated procreation as one of man's most fundamental rights, but analysis cannot stop here. It has long been established that no right, no matter how fundamental, is absolute. This is true even when the rights involved are specifically guaranteed by the Bill of Rights. For example, even in the First Amendment area the Court has never held the freedom of speech and press to be inviolate. To the contrary, the ambit of the First Amendment rights has been limited on many occasions.

PROCREATION: NOT AN UNLIMITED RIGHT OR ABSOLUTELY PROTECTED INTEREST

In *Skinner,* the Court struck down an Oklahoma law requiring the sterilization of a person convicted three times of a felony involving moral turpitude. The statutory scheme exempted from sterilization those convicted of "offenses arising out of the violation of the prohibitory laws, revenue acts, embezzlement, or political offenses." Justice Douglas, in the majority opinion, coined the phrase "invidious discrimination," thereby charting a new path for equal protection analysis, while at the same time he mapped a new course for due process considerations. Concerning the equal protection argument, *Skinner* was the first case to afford "strict scrutiny."

"Strict scrutiny" would dictate that if a classification discriminates with respect to a right of very great importance, it is not to be sustained merely because the classification has a rational basis for enactment. The state must provide a substantial justification for its classification and if it does not the discrimination is invidious. Even though an equal protection case, *Skinner* is often cited for the due process protection of a fundamental interest, the right to procreate, and many believe this analysis forecloses the due process issue.

It should be pointed out that although the majority observed that procreation was a "basic civil right" in the equal protection context, it was the two concurring opinions that addressed themselves to the due process analysis. Even those pronouncements were not dispositive, but only suggested possible answers. Justice Stone believed that the Oklahoma law was defective and that the real question was not equal protection but procedural due process; personal liberty was being invaded without the individual's being given an opportunity to show that his case was not within the ambit of the legislation. Justice Jackson met the due process issue straight on: "There are limits to the extent to which a legislatively represented majority may conduct biological experiments at the expense of the dignity and personality and natural powers of a minority—even those who have been guilty of what the majority define as crimes." But the Justice candidly pointed out that "this Act falls down before reaching this problem. . . ." Thus, the *Skinner* majority did not confront the due process question; the holding of the case is *not* that procreation is a fundamental due process interest. In this regard it is also important to notice that the *Skinner* Court cited with approval *Buck v. Bell,* 274 U.S. 200 (1927), a Justice Holmes opinion upholding a eugenic sterilization law as a valid exercise of the police power. They distinguished the applicability of *Buck v. Bell* because of the equal protection problems present in *Skinner*.

Given these factors, even if one assumed procreation a fundamental interest, the issue presented vis-à-vis a Population

Control Statute is not answered by *Skinner.* The Population Control Statute would not deny the right of procreation, but instead would merely limit the unbridled exercise of that right. It would be a limitation of the number of children rather than the right to have children. Indeed, in allowing children that are born to live a higher quality of life, a Population Control Statute might be considered as reaffirming an individual's fundamental right to procreate.

The critical question is this: At what point can the state, on behalf of the society, limit an individual's right to uncontrolled discretion over the size of his family? As we have seen, the right to procreate is not mentioned in the Constitution. Although procreation was held in *Skinner* to be a fundamental interest protected by the Fourteenth Amendment's equal protection demand of "strict scrutiny" in judicial review, whether procreation is a due process right emanating from, as Justice Douglas has indicated in other contexts, the fringes of the various provisions of the Bill of Rights has not been considered. Furthermore, even if procreation is a due process right, whether the limitation on the number of children born to an individual will be afforded similar constitutional footing is a question still to be decided. It is at least arguable that once an individual has had a certain number of children, the right to have more children is no longer a fundamental interest.

"MARITAL PRIVACY": A DISTINCTION AND MANY DIFFERENCES

A "marital privacy" argument against a Population Control Statute requires analysis of the Court's holding in *Griswold v. Connecticut,* 381 U.S. 479 (1965). This case presents a clash of judicial philosophies regarding the due process clause of the Fourteenth Amendment. The long-debated issue is whether fundamental rights, not specifically enumerated in the first eight amendments, are afforded protection from state action under that amendment's due process clause. This question, along with the closely related issue of the applicable standard of judicial review, has been the source of continuing dispute among members of the Court.

Notwithstanding these warring judicial philosophies, the *Griswold* Court struck down a Connecticut statute that prohibited the use of contraceptive devices. Petitioners were a licensed physician and a Yale Medical School professor. Both gave birth control information, instruction, and medical advice to married persons. They had examined women and prescribed the best contraceptive device for their use. Fees were usually charged, though some couples paid nothing. Justice Douglas, in delivering the opinion of the Court, held that marital privacy is protected under the Bill of Rights and thus the statute infringing upon that privacy was unconstitutional. He asserted that "zones of privacy" are created by the First, Fourth, Fifth and Ninth Amendments. It is the sum of these "penumbras" that gives rise to the concept of marital privacy.

Justice Black, in a concurring opinion in the same case, called Douglas' decision the "natural law—due process" view. In contrast to Douglas, Black has been called the chief proponent of the doctrine of "absolute incorporation." Black's theory was that the Fourteenth Amendment applies only the Bill of Rights to the states. There is no basis for "judicial creation" of fundamental rights outside those enumerated in the first eight amendments. Accordingly, it is the Court's duty to protect the rights specifically guaranteed in the Constitution, but not to pass judgment on the reasonableness of state or federal statutes which might impair unenumerated rights.

At first it might seem that Black's strict incorporation view would be more favorable to enactment of a Population Control Statute. Since the right to procreate is not specifically mentioned in the first eight amendments, Black's theory would not protect it. But the Constitution's broad Fifth Amendment guarantee of "due process" could be utilized to invalidate legislation. A justice could employ Black's strict incorporation test to reach a result identical to "natural law" due process. Therefore, although the philosophies seem far apart, they may be two different modes for development of a similar plan of constitutional rights.

Justice Goldberg, concurring specially, addressed the issue of a Population Control Statute in *Griswold* dictum by asserting: "Surely the Government, *absent a showing of a compelling subordinating state interest,* could not decree that all husbands and wives must be sterilized after two children have been born to them" (emphasis added). Even the highblown rehetoric of the Justice cannot mask the flexibility of an otherwise seemingly caustic remark that ". . . the showing of a compelling. . . state interest" could justify the enactment of a compulsory sterilization statute.

Ultimately, even the *Griswold* opinion, thought by some to foreclose any possible restrictions on the marital relation, is not an absolute. Whatever would be required to show a compelling state interest, it seems that the mood of the country at the time of legislative enactment would be a factor in determining whether the interest were present. Were the nation to change its disposition with regard to population control, showing a compelling state interest would be less difficult.

Additionally, the thrust of *Griswold,* while under the guise of marital privacy, is to foster contraception and the control of the "unwanted birth." This factor should be analyzed by those who would cite *Griswold* as a case ending debate on a Population Control Statute. One equally sensible approach to *Griswold* is to see it as an attempt by the Court to encourage voluntary means of population control. In any event, whether "marital privacy" would prevent the enactment of a Population Control Statute was not considered. Moreover, while today's methods of contraception may involve a disruption of marital privacy, methods which science has nearly perfected for contraception are arguably outside the area which arose in *Griswold.* It is difficult to envision how a polio-type sugar cube taken once every five years and which was entirely reversible upon taking another capsule could be considered an invasion of marital privacy.

THE POLICE POWER AND INVASION OF THE BODY: THE COMPULSORY VACCINATION CASES

Another argument that might be raised against a Population Control Statute is that the act of sterilization is an invasion of the body that exceeds the police power of the state, and is foreign to the mores of Western government. However, the continuing validity of compulsory vaccination statutes in the early smallpox cases and more recently in the polio context suggests that the state's responsibility in protecting the public health and safety of its citizens could provide the police power rationale for the legislative enactment of a Population Control Statute.

Jacobson v. Massachusetts, 197 U.S. 11 (1905) challenged a compulsory vaccination ordinance that would bear a great deal of similarity to a Population Control Statute. At the turn of this century the State of Massachusetts had authorized local government bodies to pass compulsory vaccination laws. Pursuant to the state statute, the City of Cambridge passed an ordinance that required all individuals over the age of twenty-one either to be vaccinated or to pay a five dollar fine. The defendant refused to be vaccinated and was prosecuted. Part of the defense was that the statute interfered with the control of one's body. The Supreme Court in 1905 upheld the conviction and the ordinance on the ground that the state statute was a reasonable exercise of the police power in an attempt to protect public health.

In underscoring the fact that no right is absolute, the Court emphasized that no one can act freely if that action would harm or damage another. As the Court stated: "Even liberty itself, the greatest of all rights, is not an unrestricted license to act according to one's own will. It is only freedom from restraint under conditions essential to the equal enjoyment of the same rights by others. It is, then, liberty regulated by law." Explicit was the notion that one's relationship to others might require a limitation on the exercise of those rights, as well as a recognition of the individual's rights. The concept of a "compelling state interest" is closely tied to this notion of individual rights and the dictates of the state, and was utilized in *Jacobson* before its doctrinal formulation in later caselaw. According to the Court:

> There is, of course, a sphere within which the individual may assert the supremacy of his own will and rightfully dispute the authority of any human government, especially of any free government existing under a written constitution, to interfere with the exercise of that will. But it is equally true that in every well-ordered society charged with the duty of conserving the safety of its members the rights of the individual in respect of his liberty may at times, under the pressure of great dangers, be subjected to such restraint, to be enforced by reasonable regulations, as the safety of the general public may demand.

Thus, the Court in *Jacobson* utilized the compelling state interest test years before its doctrinal formulation.

Justice Holmes extended *Jacobson* in *Buck v. Bell*, 274 U.S. 200 (1927), relying on it for the amazing proposition that "the principle that sustains compulsory vaccination is broad enough to cover cutting the Fallopian tubes." Juxtaposed to the *Buck* statement is the idea that there are areas in which a state (police power or not) cannot work its dictates against the will of a sovereign people; no doubt population control does raise the spectre of a 1984 world in the minds of many.

2. Equal Protection Roadblocks

The Fourteenth Amendment guarantee of equal protection forms the basis of another possible objection to a compulsory sterilization statute. Although *Griswold* was decided on due process grounds, it has been suggested that an equal protection rationale may have been more appropriate. *Skinner,* as we have seen, was an equal protection case, though usually cited for the proposition that procreation is a fundamental right guaranteed by the due process clause. In recent years the reach of equal protection has been greatly expanded, and so discussion may focus on the relevance of recent developments in the law of equal protection. Indeed, these developments may signal not only a future decline in the Court's receptibility to equal protection cases but also a change in the scope of review for equal protection cases. First, it must be noted that if a compelling state interest could overcome due process objections, it surely could cure equal protection problems. Second, the Supreme Court's decision in *Dandridge v. Williams,* 397 U.S. 471 (1970) may indicate a retreat from the former standard of "strict scrutiny" in judicial review. According to *Dandridge,* if a statutory scheme can be characterized as involving an "economic-social" matter, rather than a fundamental human right, the lower standard of review, the "any rational basis" test is applicable. It certainly can be argued that legislation limiting family size does not involve a fundamental human right or interest but instead an economic and social issue. This argument seems particularly appealing because the criteria employed for distinguishing between a fundamental constitutional right or interest and a concern of an economic and social nature is not now clear.

Conceptionally it does not seem that equal protection could forever block legislation. Nonetheless, objections of the black race to the Population Control Statute would raise an interesting equal protection problem. Their charge would be voiced in terms of "genocide." The question would involve the constitutionality of a Population Control Statute's percentage freeze of blacks in the population. However, since equal protection analysis implicitly suggests that statutory redrafting should be a solution to any "invidious discrimination," their argument misses the thrust of the equal protection clause of the Fourteenth Amendment. Indeed, if a "compelling state interest" could be shown, a Population Control Statute would be immune from blacks' equal protection challenge. But even if less than a compelling state interest were demonstrated, needed legislation might not be stopped on equal protection grounds. First, the Court could adopt a position that a compelling state interest was not required because "economic-social" legislation was involved. Second, though no precedent exists for this solution, the black growth rate could be analyzed, a future black growth rate projected, and a certain number of black families then allowed to have more than two children. Third, the Court might embrace a new middle ground standard of review in equal protection cases.

THE RISE AND FALL OF EQUAL PROTECTION

Recently, the doctrinal analysis advanced in *Skinner v. Oklahoma,* 316 U.S. 536 (1942) was applied in *Shapiro v. Thompson,* 394 U.S. 618 (1969). In *Shapiro,* the one-year residency requirement in state welfare laws was held invalid on equal protection grounds. The Court pointed out that the residency requirement was a classification that transgressed a constitutionally protected interest, that of one's right to travel from state to state, although no particular constitutional provision was relied upon. Because the classification infringed upon a fundamental interest, the discrimination was invidious and unconstitutional unless it was necessary to promote a compelling governmental interest. While there might have been a rational basis for the classification, this mere showing of a rational relationship between the required residency period and the objectives of the state in requiring the waiting period was not sufficient to justify the classification.

The Court was not persuaded by arguments advanced in support of a valid governmental interest in setting a residency waiting period. Disapproved were arguments that the state might seek to limit those indigents from other states who sought larger benefits or to limit its expenditures. Other governmental aims were recognized as establishing a "rational basis" for the statute's enactment. It was argued that certain administrative and related governmental objectives were helped by the waiting period requirement; the one-year requirement:

1. facilitates the planning of the welfare budget;
2. provides an objective test of residency,
3. minimizes the opportunity for recipients fraudulently to receive payments from more than one jurisdiction; and
4. encourages early entry of new residents into the labor force.

These arguments were cited by the Court as "a mere showing of a rational relationship between the waiting period and these four admittedly permissible state objectives," but they fell short of compelling state interest criteria.

According to some, the *Shapiro* case was the logical extension of the invidious discrimination rationale delineated in *Skinner*. If this is so, then the inquiry might be reduced to a three-part test. In an adjudication employing this "strict scrutiny" test, the Court must decide, first, whether the classification results in discrimination against a disadvantaged group, and, second, whether the discrimination relates to a fundamental interest. If both these questions are answered affirmatively, the burden rests upon the state to justify its classification by proof of a compelling state interest.

But *Shapiro* had been law less than a year when *Dandridge v. Williams,* placed large question marks around the continuing validity of its equal protection rationale and the "strict scrutiny" concept for certain nonsocial discriminations. In fact, *Dandridge* may have been the beginning of a retreat by the Court from a compelling state interest test in equal protection cases. The new test, signaling the decline of "substantive equal protection," might be a modified rational basis test. The argument for extending active judicial review or strict scrutiny to equal protection cases is that certain disadvantaged "suspect groups" (women, illegitimates) have little or no political strength. While this argument has appeal, the potential stretch of the disadvantaged group aspect of an equal protection test is infinite. By definition, every loser in the legislative process is a minority or potentially classifiable as "disadvantaged."

Dandridge indicates that the Court may no longer be willing to extend the scope of "strict scrutiny" in equal protection cases beyond racial classifications and constitutionally guaranteed rights. As happened in the late 1930s in the context of allowing needed New Deal recovery programs to move forward, judicial restraint would be manifested through a "restrained standard of review." In those years entire areas of law formerly believed constitutionally prohibited by substantive economic due process were upheld. Applying this narrower standard of equal protection, in *Dandridge,* the Court upheld, by a 5-3 vote, the validity of Maryland's maximum welfare grant regulation. The regulation limited total state Aid for Dependent Children (AFDC) assistance to a monthly $250 per family. As a result, larger families did not receive an amount equivalent to their needs, while smaller families did. Since this might discourage a welfare recipient from having a large family, one might say that the Court in *Dandridge* upheld the validity of an incentive to hold down population.

Writing for the majority, Justice Stewart reasoned that since the maximum grant regulation was of a "social and economic nature," it would be viewed under the more traditional, restrained equal protection review. According to the Justice, the rational basis standard of review is a standard that is true to the principle that the Fourteenth Amendment gives the federal courts no power to impose upon the states their view of what constitutes wise economic or social policy.

The Court found Maryland's maximum grant system supportable on four grounds:

1. in terms of legitimate state interests in encouraging gainful employment,
2. in maintaining an equitable balance in economic status between welfare families and those supported by a wage earner,
3. in providing incentives for family planning,
4. in allocating public funds in such a way as fully to meet the needs of the largest possible number of families.

In answering the district court's opinion that the Maryland regulation was "invalid on its face for overreaching," the Court pointed out,

For this Court to approve the invalidation of state economic or social regulation as "overreaching" would be far too reminiscent of an era when the Court thought the Fourteenth Amendment gave it power to strike down state laws, "because they may be unwise, improvident, or out of harmony with a particular school of thought." That era long ago passed into history.

How can *Dandridge* be reconciled with *Shapiro?* Justice Marshall, dissenting, felt that the Court should not apply different standards of review simply because an interest is classified as either "fundamental" or "economic." Instead, according to Marshall, the Court should balance the state's interest in each challenged statute against the individual's need for benefit. The Court in *Shapiro* struck down the one-year residency requirement because it was a classification that infringed a fundamental interest, the right to travel interstate. In *Dandridge,* it upheld the Maryland maximum welfare grant statute as being merely economic and social legislation. But, assuming that other states have no maximum grant provisions, the welfare residents of those states who desire to move to Maryland will also be impaired in the exercise of their fundamental right to travel from state to state.

An explanation for this incongruity is possible. *Dandridge* may be the harbinger of change in the equal protection area. The Court may believe that it was in error in initially extending "strict scrutiny" beyond those rights explicitly guaranteed by the Constitution. It might not only refuse to expand the circle of fundamental interests already created by the doctrine of "substantive equal protection," but also contract those fundamental interests that have been judicially created.

There seem to be two reasons for stepping back to a rational basis test in equal protection analysis. First, it is conceptually difficult, if not impossible, to limit the extension of "other fundamental interests demanding strict scrutiny." It is hard to find a state law that could not be seen as classifying with regard to either the fundamental right to travel interstate or another fundamental interest, such as wealth. Surely all these laws cannot be unconstitutional. Second, the Supreme Court, a basically "anti-majoritarian" institution, must attempt to reconcile the Fourteenth Amendment's command of equal protection with the long-standing idea that in a democratic society the legislature rather than the judiciary is responsible for allocating not only the benefits, but also the burdens of a governmental structure. One method the Court has for mediating these two competing interests is the employment of two standards of review. Now, perhaps, a third standard is needed.

Under the rational basis test, a court would overturn a legislature's classification only when that classification is so palpably arbitrary that the court could not conceive of any constitutionally allowable objective which is rationally related. In reality, this standard of "restrained review" may amount to abandoning all but the most superficial review.

However, when a constitutional right or a fundamental personal right is involved, the Court will review the classification more carefully, demanding a convincing demonstration that it possesses a close relationship to the statutory schema. The required level of precision is unclear. In fact, it may vary according to the importance of the personal interests involved. If a fundamental constitutional right of protected interest is involved, a state must first use the least onerous means in accomplishing its objective. Further, even if the classification is well suited to achieve its objective, the legislation may fail unless it serves a state interest that "overrides" the personal interests involved. In other words, a "compelling state interest" must be shown.

With regard to a Population Control Statute, after *Dandridge,* the Supreme Court could classify such a statute as "economic and social" legislation, and therefore could require only a "rational basis" to sustain its constitutionality. This restrained standard of review would exemplify the "strict constructionism" of the Burger Court that *Dandridge* may be signaling.

Another solution would be for the Court to create a third test in cases involving fundamental rights. Occupying the middle ground between the extremes of the "compelling state interest" and the "any rational basis" test, a new formulation, "urgent and convincing," might be advanced. Under this test, the legislature would be required, first, to demonstrate that the need for the proposed legislation is urgent, and second, to show that there is more than just "any rational basis" for its enactment. If this were done, the Court need not require a compelling state interest. If the new test were applied, a legislature that held extensive investigations and hearings before the passing of a Population Control Statute would have little problem in making the required showings.

But even if the Court were to apply "strict scrutiny" to a Population Control Statute, analysis could sustain its constitutionality provided it were shown that the statute employed the least onerous means of limiting population, and that the control of population was indeed a "compelling state interest" which could justify limiting family size.

3. The Least Onerous Alternative Principle

Another objection that might be voiced against a Population Control Statute is that the statute was not the "least onerous alternative" open to a government bent on controlling population growth. The doctrine of the least onerous alternative helps to answer this objection. Going back to its philosophical origins, the doctrine balances a state's police-power basis for enacting legislation against the citizens' constitutionally protected bundle of rights. As already pointed out, few rights, including those of the Bill of Rights, are absolute when they encounter a "subordinating and compelling state interest." On the other hand, the citizen does have rights against the oppressive and unnecessary exercise of governmental police power.

The following hypothetical demonstrates the operation of the "least onerous alternative doctrine": A state has a desired legislative goal X, here, the control of population growth. To achieve goal X, the legislature enacts law A, a Population Control Statute that requires compulsory sterilization of one parent after the birth of two children to a family unit. Law A is attacked on the grounds that it constitutes either an unconstitutional deprivation of due process or is invalid under the equal protection clause. Were the issue to come before the Court, and if it could be shown that there existed "less onerous means" of achieving goal X, namely law B, then law A would be held unconstitutional. This determination operates irrespective of showing a compelling state interest.

The judicial doctrine that a government must employ the legislative course least restrictive of individual rights consistent with accomplishing a desired legislative end arose in the economic regulation cases, and has spread to other constitutionally protected rights. In the *Griswold* case, three of the four majority opinions made reference to the least onerous alternative principle. As Justice Douglas stated, "A governmental purpose to control or prevent activities constitutionally subject to state regulation may not be achieved by means which sweep unnecessarily broadly and thereby invade the area of protected freedoms." Accordingly, a constitutional analysis involving a Population Control Statute must consider the available less onerous alternatives.

Nonetheless, there are two interrelated criticisms of the least onerous alternative principle as a tool for striking down legislation. First, the determination of whether a particular piece of legislation is the least onerous alternative requires factual inquiries and legislative analysis. There is the question concerning whether this inquiry is an appropriate role for the Court and the judicial system. Historically, courts and commentators have frowned on attempts to enlarge judicial inquiry into what have been termed "legislative facts." The inherent limitations of a court as a fact-finding body make the judiciary a less-well-suited institution for finding these facts. However, the Court must consider, *sub silentio,* "legislative facts" in any interest-balancing test it attempts. With this reality in view, it is no longer as disturbing to find the adjudication of "legislative facts" taking place in a judicial context. A second major objection to the least onerous alternative formulation is that the Court, by indicating the alternatives available, is "legislating." Although the Court has refused to specify alternatives in recent cases, the spectre of its acting as a "super-legislature" remains.

TODAY'S LESS ONEROUS ALTERNATIVES

There are at present less onerous alternatives of controlling population. Voluntary sterilization could be encouraged by legislative enactments making available population control devices and techniques. Further, appropriate statutes could repeal present laws that inhibit voluntary population control, such as those limiting the right to abortion, voluntary sterilization, and the advertising, dissemination, or use of birth control information, devices, and drugs.

Having eliminated obstacles to voluntary control, the government could initiate programs to foster voluntary contraception without providing direct monetary incentives. Government-funded centers could be set up to provide free counseling and free contraceptives. Abortions and sterilizations could be offered free to all. These services might be made available either through present private means or through a newly organized system of paramedical personnel trained in the simple procedures of birth control and abortion. In fact, to carry the program to its logical completion, the effort could be placed under control of an independent agency or become a cabinet level department. Finally, since much present television programming encourages child-bearing, the federal communications "fairness doctrine" could be interpreted to require radio and television to devote time to programs discouraging large families.

Assuming the failure of proposals outlined above, the government might attempt to induce lower levels of population through economic incentives. First, cash payments could be given to individuals willing to undergo sterilization. Second, an annual subsidy could be paid to each woman of child-bearing age who did not give birth during the year. Third, the tax laws could be revised; sections that act as incentives to having large families could be repealed by code sections that encourage reductions in family size.

The validity of cash payments and subsidies is doubtful under the equal protection clause of the Constitution. These two programs would necessarily have a greater effect on the poor, and since a fundamental right is infringed, an argument similar to that which we encountered concerning a Population Control Statute prevails. The difference is that the use of direct monetary incentives seems a much clearer violation of the equal protection clause. A Population Control Statute, on the other hand, affects each family unit identically; each is limited to two children. However, direct monetary incentives clearly classify on the basis of wealth.

A similar equal protection criticism is applicable to tax incentives, although the revision of tax laws may present different considerations. Recently there have been introduced measures which would modify income tax exemptions to favor small families.

Finally, there are alternative compulsory measures. Compulsory abortion could be demanded of a woman already having two children. Aside from the obvious administrative difficulties, women, as a suspect classification entitled to equal protection, might successfully argue that they were bearing the brunt of punishment—the abortion—while the men were left untouched. Moreover, compulsory abortion might be considered even more repugnant than compulsory sterilization.

4. The Compelling State Interest

The least onerous alternative bears a close relation to the determination of a compelling state interest. In fact when the Court holds that no compelling state interest exists, it might be shorthand for acknowledging the existence of a less onerous alternative. Indeed, the possibility of a less onerous alternative may rob the legislature of a compelling state interest, and the ultimate determination of a less onerous alternative remains a function of the strength of the compelling state interest.

Where constitutional rights and fundamental interests are threatened, a state must carry the burden of proving that its action is justified by a "compelling subordinating state interest." The constitutionality of such enactment is not presumed, and a heavy burden of justification is placed on the state which desires the legislation upheld. Though the doctrine has been used to strike down many legislative enactments, exact definition of a compelling state interest has been attempted by few commentators. But regardless of definitional difficulties, some enactments would always remain beyond governmental control. In economic regulation, the sudden death of substantive due process demonstrates that exigencies of the times will bear heavily on the Court's decisions. In that area, statutes that were classed as blatantly unconstitutional thirty-five or forty years ago are today unquestioned. Who can foretell what governmental action may be required in the next fifty years? And in this determination, what help is the label "compelling state interest?"

The cases of federal enactments sustained upon a showing of a compelling state interest are few and no clear "test" emerges from them. However, it is important to recognize that the Court is balancing the importance of the governmental interest against the gravity of harm to the individual's civil liberties.

DETERMINING A COMPELLING STATE INTEREST

Before passage of a Population Control Statute, a legislature would complete an extensive fact-finding inquiry to determine whether compulsory sterilization was required to limit population growth. There would have to be a determination that the state must prevent individuals from exercising their "liberty" in unlimited procreation in order to maintain the "liberty" of other individuals in the society. Ultimately, the freedom that is preserved might increase the overall well-being of the human species, manifested by a richer and less polluted environment, and a higher requisite share of scarce public and free goods. A compelling state interest in restraining the individual's present procreative freedom would have to be shown. In determining whether that compelling state interest burden had been sustained, the Court would be required to engage in legislative fact-finding.

Although it is not clear what scientific evidence would have to be presented to prove a compelling state interest, an attempt to pinpoint some necessary evidence would be useful. Certainly, statistics should be analyzed and the views of scientists assimilated so as to appraise not only the present but also the future status of a "compelling state interest" test.

Nonetheless, one fact is clear, a population problem does exist. Recently there have been detailed analyses of the various authorities and available scientific data about the problem. While a detailed, analytic legislative determination would be in order, extensive inquiry is beyond the scope of this article.

The traditional view was that the only justification for population control would be the inability of the United States to support its population. This was the "population explosion" question of the 1960s and its concern was food scarcity. More recently, inquiry about the quality of the American physical and social environment has drawn attention. In addition, serious doubt has been cast upon our society's ability to continue to consume massive amounts of raw materials during the "shortages of the 70s." Vis-à-vis population control these issues are fundamental, for they bring to light a critical distinction between man and animal that has often been overlooked. Man's most fundamental talent is his ability to use his brain and imagination through law—to change, to shape, and to improve his environs. Animals are left to the Darwinian "law of the jungle" for their well-being. To say to mankind that it is deprived of the right to shape the environment might be considered the denial of a right at least as fundamental as procreation. It is the right of mankind to determine the nature and quality of its future existence.

Whatever the rationale behind population control, it seems that most have accepted the goal of reducing "replacement fertility" from the present rate of "about three" to two. "Replacement fertility" is the average number of children born to a couple in each generation. Given the present age distribution, even if the average "replacement fertility" were reduced to 2.1 in 1975, the population would not stop growing until 2040. Meanwhile, the population would have grown another 35 to 40 percent, reaching a figure of 290 million. That growth would occur even if action were taken immediately to decrease "fertility replacement." In light of this built-in time lag on growth stoppage, the legislature may determine it is now time to act.

The heart of the dilemma is that while most believe some kind of curb on population growth is necessary, not everyone can agree on the means to accomplish it. Many favor voluntary means of easing growth. Such attempts are admirable, but, at this point, likely to be futile.

The President's Commission on Population Growth espoused the voluntary approach. The Commission's focus was on "unwanted births" and the use of liberalized abortion to slow growth. In response, it has been argued that recommendations aimed at "unwanted births" will not work, or will bring results too insignificant to be helpful. While it is too soon to determine who is right, and those who urge compulsory measures could be wrong, a legislature may determine that voluntary means are too little too late. At that point, the Court will be forced to decide whether compulsory legislations could withstand a constitutional test. The Court, in evaluating a Population Control Statute, may find it useful to examine eugenic sterilization.

THE PRECEDENT OF EUGENIC STERILIZATION

Sterilization as a birth control method is not a new development. In the early 1900s many states passed compulsory eugenic sterilization laws to prevent designated persons from procreating.

The Pennsylvania Legislature in 1905 was the first state assembly to pass a sterilization bill. The purpose of the bill was prevention of idiocy through the sterilization of institutionalized "idiots." However, the bill was vetoed by the Governor. Indiana was first to enact a sterilization statute; the state supreme court held it unconstitutional. It was not until 1925 that the Michigan and Virginia courts upheld the validity of their sterilization statutes. The Virginia decision was appealed to the United States Supreme Court.

Buck v. Bell, 274 U.S. 200 (1927), a case known most for Justice Holmes' caustic remark, "three generations of imbeciles are enough," involved Carrie Buck, a feeble-minded woman, who was committed to the State Colony for Epileptics and Feeble-minded. Carrie was not only the daughter of a feeble-minded mother but also the mother of a feeble-minded illegitimate child. The state had ordered her sterilized and the Virginia Court had held that Carrie Buck "is the probable potential parent of socially inadequate offspring, likewise afflicted, that she may be sexually sterilized without detriment to her general health and that her welfare and that of society will be promoted by her sterilization." She claimed the sapingectomy authorized by statute was a violation of her constitutional right of bodily integrity and therefore violated the due process clause of the Fourteenth Amendment. The Court per Justice Holmes reasoned that Ms. Buck's interest was outweighed by the paramount state interest.

> We have seen more than once that the public welfare may call upon the best citizens for their lives. It would be strange if it could not call upon those who already sap the strength of the State for these lesser sacrifices, often not felt to be such by those concerned, in order to prevent our being swamped with incompetence. It is better for all the world, if instead of waiting to execute the degenerate offspring for crime, or to let them starve for their imbecility, society can prevent those who are manifestly unfit from continuing their kind. The principle that sustains compulsory vaccination is broad enough to cover cutting the Fallopian tubes. Three generations of imbeciles are enough.

After that decision, twenty-nine states passed eugenic sterilization laws which contain provisions for the sterilization of mental defectives already institutionalized in state facilities; not all require the consent of the person to be sterilized. In the last few years we have read about cases where persons were sterilized without giving consent. In some cases, consent has been forced upon the young or coupled with the threat of losing welfare funds if the person resisted sterilization.

THE RATIONALE AND CRITICISM OF EUGENIC STERILIZATION: THE POSSIBLE RELEVANCE TO COMPULSORY STERILIZATION

The historical sketch above vividly indicates that the idea of compulsory sterilization as a means of birth control is not a modern innovation. It also indicates that in certain instances the right to procreate is not absolute. Procreation may have to yield when a stronger state interest is presented. Furthermore, the courts in eugenic sterilization cases have consistently held that the state interest outweighs the interest of the individual.

The state interest most often advanced to justify eugenic sterilization is the improvement of the human species, or alternatively, the prevention of the species' deterioration. Feeble-mindedness, insanity, epilepsy, and other designated traits are viewed as inheritable characteristics to be controlled lest the nation be filled with incompetents who would tax already limited state resources. This premise has been questioned by critics who claim that medical knowledge of heredity has not yet reached the point where such a positive assertion can be made. Though this is a valid criticism of eugenic sterilization, the narrow issue of heredity is irrelevant to a Population Control Statute. The transferability of human traits is no longer in question. Without exception, everyone who falls within the terms of the statute would be sterilized.

The scientific inquiry most relevant to population control focuses on simple geometric increases in population and asks simply how much time we have. While the eugenics problems could afford to wait a scientific solution to the question of trait transmissibility, population control advocates are unable to allow mankind the luxury of awaiting a scientific answer, because of the grave consequences likely to flow from the time lag. Without eugenic sterilization additional feeble-minded persons would be born, but many believe that this possibility does not justify sterilization and that we can afford to wait. In the Population Control situation the total breakdown of society and the destruction of mankind as we know it could result from an insufficient supply of food and mineral resources. The Arab oil boycott and the "shortages of the 70s" foretell this possibility. We may not be allowed the luxury of watchful waiting. Whether we can afford to delay will depend upon an intelligent evaluation of available scientific evidence.

Eugenic sterilization critics also fear that the logic behind the statutes might be used to extend the class of persons sterilized. They point to an early Model Eugenic Sterilization Statute as evidence of this danger. This 1922 model law included the feeble-minded, the insane, the criminal (including the delinquent and wayward), the epileptic, the inebriate (including habitual drug users), the diseased (including the tuberculous, the syphilitics, the leprous and others with chronic, infectious, and legally separable diseases), the blind and deaf, the deformed (including crippled), and the dependents (which included orphans, ne'er-do-wells, homeless, tramps, and paupers). In addition, the opponents of the Statute indicate that there may be a danger of racial discrimination. Discretionary elements pervade the eugenics laws. First, there is legislative discretion in designating which class of persons can be sterilized: the feeble-minded, epileptics, insane. Second, there is room for discretion within the class since most statutes empower the director of a state institution to initiate proceedings against an inmate whom he deems likely to produce children with undesirable traits. Third, most states provide Eugenic Boards with power to determine whether an operation should be performed. Hence, though the determination is appealable, there is room for abuse, whether racial or otherwise, on at least three levels. The Population Control Statute provides no element of discretion since all who have had two children must be sterilized. This makes abuse unlikely in the compulsory sterilization context.

Finally, critics of eugenic sterilization have questioned Justice Holmes' analogy in *Buck v. Bell* between compulsory vaccination and eugenic sterilization. According to Justice Holmes in *Buck,* both vaccination and sterilization involve an invasion of the body to promote the welfare of both the individual and that of society. With vaccination, the direct and immediate benefit to the individual is immunity from the disease. For society there is less danger of an epidemic. But critics point out that in the eugenics case the benefit to the individual is difficult to find. Similarly one might argue that in the population control case, the individual may not derive the immediate "vaccination" benefit.

However, further examination indicates that Holmes' analysis is correct and that the individual will be rewarded in both the eugenic and compulsory sterilization situations. After eugenics, fewer feeble-minded people will occupy institutions and therefore more of the state's scarce resources can be spent on the sterilized individual's welfare. Indeed, this resources argument has been advanced to support most eugenics programs. *A fortiori,* a Population Control Statute not only saves scarce state resources, but also pays an ecological and social dividend. With fewer people, the individual can benefit from a higher quality in the nation's free goods—a cleaner and more abundant supply of air and water—not to mention the pleasure of "undercrowding." The society can function more productively and provide a higher standard of life for each human being.

The validity of scientific assertions concerning the quality of life and the possible adverse effects of inaction would be a large aspect of preenactment legislative determination. But once a legislature determined upon a "valid and compelling showing" that the societal choice was population limitation through compulsory sterilization, the Court might have to determine the statute's constitutionality. Perhaps, as Holmes suggested, "the answer is that the law does all that is needed when it does all that it can." At least, the precedent of eugenic sterilization remains—sterile for the moment, but ready at any time to be pressed in service should the need require it.

Conclusion

When the question of enacting a Population Control Statute (compulsory sterilization after two children) is placed starkly before the American people, there is bound to be active and vigorous discussion. In debate involving emotionally charged issues, arguments are often reduced to Biblical quotations. Such sayings, although devoid of theoretical and logical support, often are used not only to shore up a weak argument but also to characterize a strong one. Opponents of compulsory sterilization, arguing the freedom of the individual to choose and the fundamental nature of the right of procreation, might seize on the admonition, "Be fruitful and multiply" (Genesis 1:28). Indeed, even without the Bible, their arguments concerning individual freedom would be powerful. This article has recognized that there are strong arguments in support of a Population Control Statute. In that regard, but of more psychological than logical utility, the Biblical quotations to which proponents of population control can refer is Romans 13:1-2: "Everyone must obey the state authorities; for no authority exists without God's permission, and the existing authorities have been put there by God. Whoever opposes the existing authority opposes what God has ordered; and anyone who does so will bring judgment on himself." This may be the Biblical counterpart of the Court's "compelling state interest" doctrine.

With regard to constitutional questions, one should recognize that the entire constitutional rights and protected interests analysis should be seen as a shell game the Court must play in adapting to the changing mores and demands of modern urban society, without violating certain rights, reserved in the people, which cannot be infringed upon by the government. The central issue is to determine which of these rights will remain beyond government control.

Focusing on the fundamental interests, procreation and marital privacy, our analysis has considered due process and equal protection challenges to the statute. We have seen that a sterilization statute limiting a couple to two children could be constitutionally sustained through limiting *Skinner's* ambit and distinguishing *Griswold's* applicability. The notion of the appropriate standard of review and the "compelling state interest" loom undeveloped and are fundamental to this analysis. In addition, the police power rationale of the compulsory vaccination and eugenic sterilization cases may serve as precedent for sustaining a legislative scheme of compulsory sterilization.

The compelling state interest concept, along with undecided issues concerning the fundamental relationship of the individual to the government are critical to analysis of a Population Control Statute's propriety. In this context the constitutional principle of the least onerous alternative is important and may serve to postpone the Court's ultimate decision. Indeed, it is possible that a panoply of less onerous measures could blunt the sterilization issue. The ultimate question is what limit man will place upon himself in coping with the complex problems of an overpopulated country while still maintaining a high degree of individual freedom.

The thesis of this article is that sterilization is a viable answer to population control. It suggests that a Population Control Statute could be sustained after thorough fact-finding has demonstrated that the need for compulsory sterilization is urgent and compelling. Having made that determination, the Court, utilizing the new "urgent and compelling" standard of review, could hold that unlimited procreation is not a due process right. *Dandridge* and the "strict constructionism" of the Burger Court may portend this new test. Or while upholding a fundamental interest in procreation, the Court could decline a review, relying on the legislative's "urgent and compelling" determination that a limitation of procreation is essential. Alternatively, utilizing the precedent of eugenic sterilization and the compulsory vaccination "police power" rationale, the Court could sustain the government on compelling state interest grounds.

In sum, the passage of a compulsory sterilization statute is not a mystical or academic exercise. Rather, it may be part of the cold reality of living in the last quarter of the twentieth century.

16

Involuntary Fertility Control

Paul R. and Anne H. Ehrlich

The third approach to population control is that of involuntary fertility control. Several coercive proposals deserve serious consideration, mainly because we may ultimately have to resort to them unless current trends in birthrates are rapidly reversed by other means. Some involuntary measures may prove to be less repressive or discriminatory, in fact, than some of the socioeconomic measures that have been proposed.

One idea that has been seriously proposed in India is to vasectomize all fathers of three or more children. This was defeated not only on moral grounds but on practical ones as well: there simply were not enough medical personnel available even to start on the eligible candidates, let alone deal with the new recruits added each day! Massive assistance from the developed world in the form of medical and paramedical personnel, and/or a training program for local people, might put such a policy within the realm of possibility, although it still would not be very popular. But probably India's government will have to resort to some such coercive method sooner or later, unless famine, war, or disease takes the problem out of its hands. There is little time left for educational programs and social change, and the population is probably too poor for economic measures (especially penalties) to be effective.

A program of sterilizing women after their second or third child, despite the greater difficulty of the female operation, might be easier than trying to sterilize the fathers. At least this would be the case in countries where the majority of babies are born in maternity hospitals and clinics, and where the medical corps is adequate. The problem of finding and identifying eligibles for sterilization would be simplified in this way.

The development of a sterilizing capsule that can be implanted under the skin and removed when pregnancy is desired opens another possibility for coercive control. The capsule could be implanted at puberty and might be removable, with official permission, for a limited number of births. Various approaches to administering this system have been offered, including one by economist Kenneth Boulding of the University of Colorado. His proposal is to issue to each woman at marriage a marketable license that would entitle her to a given number of children. Under such a system the number could be two if the society desired to reduce the population size slowly. To maintain a steady size, perhaps one out of four couples might be allowed to have a third child if they purchased special tickets from the government or from other women, who, having purchased them, decided not to have a child or found they had a greater need for the money. Another idea is that permission to have a third child might be granted to a limited number of couples by lottery. This system would allow governments to regulate more or less exactly the number of births over a given period of time.

Of course a government might require only implantation after childbirth. Since having a child would require positive action (removal of the capsule), many more births would be prevented than in the reverse situation. Certainly unwanted births and the problem of abortion would both be entirely avoided. The disadvantages, besides any moral objections, include the questionable desirability of having the entire female population on a continuous steroid dosage with the contingent health risks, and the logistics of implanting capsules in 50 percent of the population between the ages of fifteen and fifty.

Adding a sterilant to drinking water or staple foods is a suggestion that, initially at least, seems to horrify people more than most proposals for involuntary fertility control. Indeed this would pose some very difficult political, legal, and social questions, to say nothing of the technical problems. No such sterilant exists today. To be acceptable, such a substance would have to meet some rather stiff requirements. It would have to be uniformly effective, despite widely varying doses received by individuals, and despite varying degrees of fertility and sensitivity among individuals. It would have to be free of dangerous or unpleasant side-effects, and have no effect on members of the opposite sex, children, old people, pets, or livestock.

Botanist Richard W. Schrieber of the University of New Hampshire has proposed that a sterilizing virus could be developed, with an antidote available by injection. This would avoid the problem of finding an appropriate staple food or adjusting doses in water supplies, but it might present some other difficulties. Not the least difficulty might be the appearance of a mutant virus immune to the antidote.

Physiologist Melvin Ketchel, of the Tufts University School of Medicine, has suggested that a sterilant could be developed that would have a very specific action—for example, the prevention of implantation of the fertilized ovum. He proposed that it be used to reduce fertility levels by adjustable amounts, anywhere from 5 percent to 75 percent, rather than to sterilize the whole population completely. In this way, fertility could be adjusted from time to time to meet a society's changing needs, and there would be no need to provide an antidote. Family planning would still be needed for those couples who were highly motivated to have a small family. Subfertile and functionally sterile couples who strongly desire children could be medically assisted, as they are now, or encouraged to adopt.

This plan has the advantage of avoiding those socioeconomic programs that might tend to discriminate against particular groups in a society or that might penalize children. It would also involve no direct action against individuals, such as sterilization operations or implanted capsules. In extremely poor and overpopulated countries, such a program would undoubtedly be far more effective and far easier to administer than any of the others, at least until development and educational levels reached a point where people could be affected by small-family propaganda and be influenced by social or economic pressures. The administration of this sort of program would probably also be easier to safeguard against corruption and abuse in favor of some segments of society, although this is likely to be a problem with any form of population control, just as it is with any government program having far-reaching social consequences.

Compulsory control of family size is an unpalatable idea to many, but the alternatives may be much more horrifying. As those alternatives become clearer to an increasing number of people in the 1970s, we may well find them *demanding* such control. A far better choice, in our view, is to begin *now* with milder methods of influencing family size preferences, while ensuring that the means of birth control, including abortion and sterilization, are accessible to every human being on earth within the shortest possible time. If effective action is taken promptly, perhaps the need for involuntary or repressive measures can be averted.

Population Control and Attitudes

No form of population control, even the most coercive or repressive, will succeed for long unless individuals understand the need for it and accept the idea that humanity must limit its numbers. Therefore, the ultimate key to population control lies in changing human attitudes concerning reproductive behavior and goals in all societies. Achieving this throughout the world would be a gigantic task even if it became the world's first-priority goal, as many believe it should be.

But human survival seems certain to require population control programs, at least in some places, even before the necessary changes in attitudes can be brought about in the population. In fact, the establishment of such programs might in itself help to convince people of the seriousness of the population problem.

Most of the population control measures discussed here have never been tried; we know only that their *potential* effectiveness may be great. The socioeconomic proposals are based on knowledge of the sort of social conditions that have been associated in the past with low birth rates. We need to know more about all peoples' attitudes toward human reproduction; we need to know how these attitudes are affected by various living conditions, including some that seem virtually intolerable to us. Even more, we need to know what influences and conditions will lead to changes in these attitudes in favor of smaller families. How can we convince a poor Pakistani villager or a middle-class American that the number of children his wife bears is of crucial importance, not just to himself and his family, but also to his society? How can we make everyone care?

17

Three Phases
of Population Control

Garrett Hardin

Population control is inevitable; population control is impossible. On a spaceship, population will inevitably be controlled someday by "Nature"—by epidemics, starvation, social disorder, psychological breakdown, or some other "natural" abomination we have not yet become aware of. However, that is usually not the sort of control we have in mind when we speak of "population control"; we usually mean control by man, by human decisions. This second kind of control seems, at the moment, to be impossible—impossible because we are afraid to initiate radical change in society. We know at the outset that change will be opposed for religious, ethical, legal, political, and emotional reasons.

Population control is impossible: but we must somehow accomplish the impossible.

Who's *we*? Since we are on a spaceship, obviously "we" is everyone—all three and a half billion of us. How do you get agreement among three and a half billion people? By democratic means? How long does it take? Six hundred years? Sixteen hundred? Six thousand? We don't have that long before Nature takes over.

On a spaceship, population control will ultimately have to encompass all peoples—but not in the beginning. How could we Americans (for example) force population control on all the rest of the people in the world? By conquering them? There are seventeen times as many of them as of us. Or we might see the conflict as one of rich, industrialized countries (with a rate of increase of about 1 percent per year) versus poor and poorly

From *Exploring New Ethics for Survival* by Garrett Hardin, pp. 191-204. Copyright © 1968, 1972 by Garrett Hardin. Reprinted by permission of the author and The Viking Press, Inc.

industrialized countries (increasing at about 3 percent per year). Should the rich countries, in concert, make colonies of the poor, readopting the nineteenth-century philosophy of "the white man's burden," and forcing population control on them?

Putting aside all moral questions for the moment, who—as a purely and narrowly practical matter—would at this moment recommend such a course of action? No one, I think. Whatever our periodic lapses, we do honor the idea of national sovereignty in principle; we are not about to violate this principle and directly force population control on others. For the foreseeable future, in spite of the undeniable fact that we are all confined together in the same spaceship, the only thing a slow-breeding rich country can do is try to persuade the more populous and more rapidly breeding poor countries to slow down their breeding in order that they may increase their own rates of economic progress.

Honoring national sovereignty, we Americans can preach to the poor countries—and we no doubt shall. We will be much more effective, however, if we set an example and bring our own rate of population growth down to zero or less. How shall we do this?

Population control must be focused on women. So blunt a statement evokes cries of "Male chauvinism!" but any other approach is worse. I cannot pretend to be objective, because I am a man; but I can try to imagine myself a woman. . . . If I were a woman I would be continually running the risk of pregnancy. As a woman, I ask myself if I would trust men to take the measures required to keep *me* from getting pregnant? I answer with a resounding *No!* . . . Is that male chauvinism?

Although it takes both sexes to "create" a child, only the female can become pregnant. Biology, in effect, has made women responsible. Saddled with this inequity, women had better demand power to match their responsibility.

As the community takes over the control of population, it may be tempted to enunciate a doctrine of "joint parental responsibility" for the births that occur. The moment it enunciates a policy based on such a doctrine it will discover that it has "opened up a can of worms."

Suppose the community-decreed limit is two children per couple. How would the law respond to the problems presented by the following not unlikely cases?

1. Mary and John get divorced, after having two children. Mary takes the children. Both remarry, their new partners having had no

children previously. Suppose Mary's new husband wants a child "of his own"—can he have one? If so, Mary must exceed *her* quota. What if John's new wife wants to be a mother—is she forbidden to do so because John has twice fathered children? . . . If she promised to conceive extramaritally, would that make it all right?

2. A young woman has intercourse with several men in one month and becomes pregnant. She doesn't know who the father is, and "paternity tests," which can only *exclude* some of the candidates, do not tell us. Should each of the nonexcluded men be charged with one child? Or only a fraction of a child?

3. Five men and three women join in a group marriage. If a quota is to be assigned to the group, what should it be? $3 \times 2 = 6$? $5 \times 2 = 10$? $[(5 + 3) \div 2] \times 2 = 8$?

We haven't even considered the complications introduced by extramarital affairs, and the legal consequences of condonation. I'm afraid there are more patterns of marriage and sex than are dreamt of in Doris Day's philosophy. The law ignores this variety to its peril.

The chain of legal evidence that establishes maternity is really quite good. The evidence for paternity is always shaky, and putting a policeman under every bed really wouldn't help. "It's a wise father that knows his own child," said Shakespeare, and the science of serology hasn't changed the situation much yet.

To say that the two sexes should be equally responsible is to forget that we are not a perfectly monogamous people. Extramarital intercourse is not rare; and divorce and remarriage create what has been called "serial polygamy." If coercion is ever used in population control it will likely involve the use of sterilization. The sterilization of x men would be much less effective in reducing births than the sterilization of x women. Given a reservoir of political resistance to community control of population, one could realistically expect that even the tiniest minority of fertile men in this reservoir would be adequate to impregnate all the impregnable women in it. Many children can be produced by only a few fertile men, if fertile women seek to subvert population control.

By contrast, if women are made the target of population control, the number of children produced by the small number of women who escape the control net will, in fact, be only a small number.

I suggest that progress in controlling population within the nation will occur in three phases, which will overlap in time. These are:

1. *Voluntary phase:* the system of birth control is perfected.

2. *Educational phase:* people are persuaded to want fewer children.

3. *Coercive phase:* breeding by noncooperators (no more than a small minority of the population) is legally restricted.

To those who say the coercive phase is "unthinkable" I say *fine:* if the job can be done using only the first two approaches, there is no need to call for a third. But if the third phase is ultimately required, we had better think about it a bit beforehand.

1. Voluntary Phase

The goal of this phase is simply one of *no unwanted children.* No single *method* of birth control is foolproof, but there can be a perfect *system* of birth control. All that is necessary is that elective abortion be included in the set of methods used—as a back-up method, when other methods fail (for whatever reason). Abortion on the request of the woman can be justified as a necessity for the emancipation of women. A century ago we got rid of compulsory servitude; now we must get rid of compulsory pregnancy, and for much the same reasons.

Society has a real stake in putting an end to the birth of unwanted children. The social cost of unwanted children has been revealed by a Swedish study. For a generation Sweden has had a very slightly permissive abortion law. Most women have been denied the abortions they wanted. After more than two decades of the operation of this law, two investigators sought out children born twenty-one years earlier to mothers who had sought, but had been denied, abortions. In other words, these children were unwanted by their mothers. As young adults they were compared with others of the same age, matched carefully for area and socioeconomic status, who had presumably been wanted at the time of birth, since their mothers had not requested abortions. As compared with the controls, the unwanted children were not as healthy; they had received more psychiatric attention (presumably because it was needed); they used alcohol more; the boys had a higher rejection rate by the army; and the girls became pregnant at an earlier age.

In a welfare state everybody pays part of the cost of unwanted children. Even if society were completely indifferent to the happiness and welfare of women, it still would have ample reason to exert itself to make the system of birth control perfect. We need research to find better methods of birth control. We need to make the method we have as available as tap water to everyone everywhere, without shame. (Attempts to restrict birth control to certain ages and to the married only are sure to increase the tax burden without bringing any perceptible improvement in morality.) We still have a long way to go in the delivery of this kind of medical service (as well as others); but we are making progress.

It is unlikely that we will make a significant move into the educational phase until we recognize this hard truth:

Birth control is not population control.

Almost everybody regards the two terms as synonymous. People are encouraged in this belief by organizations that collect money for the second purpose and then use it for the first—which fails to produce the second. In India, for example, there was a gratifying increase in the use of birth control beginning in the middle of the present century; but the rate of population increase rose steadily from 1.3 percent per year in 1951 to 2.5 percent in 1968.

Why does a woman have babies? The *system* that causes women to produce babies can be analyzed into three components:

message——reception——performance

Sometimes consciously, but more often unconsciously, society exposes a woman to one message or another having to do with the desirability of her having babies, e.g., "Stop at two," or "They're cheaper by the dozen." Many different messages are bandied about.

Because "society" is an abstraction, there is some ambiguity and unclarity in the message "society" sends; or to put it another way, the reception of a message by the woman is more or less imperfect (partly because it may conflict with her preexisting desires.)

After she's received the message, her performance may not be perfectly congruent with the altered message she hears. She may decide: "no baby," but if she is using only the rhythm method to achieve this goal, assuming she has a rhythm, her performance will be only about 84 percent effective each year, on the average.

In the light of this threefold analysis of the system of population control we see why birth control is not population control. Table 1 is constructed on the assumption that a woman's reception of society's message and the performance of birth control are both perfect. Given this hypothetical perfection, population growth will be determined by the message. Let us examine some possible messages, one at a time, to see their effect. For simplicity, we assume all women marry and all women are fertile, and we ignore such complications as multiple births, infant mortality, and maternal mortality. Plugging in these variables would modify the conclusions only slightly, because they partly cancel each other out.

"Stop at two" ultimately produces a Zero Population Growth society, of course. Assuming, to begin with, that the population hasn't risen beyond a level compatible with human dignity in a spaceship, society can exist indefinitely, guided by this message.

The ZPG condition is also produced if the only message each woman receives from society is "I must have an heir," i.e., a boy. Half the women would stop breeding after having only one child, a boy. A fourth of the women would stop after having a girl, then a boy; one eighth after having girl girl boy; and so on. This *averages* two children per family (actually, slightly less, because a woman who had had, say, sixteen girls in a row might well refuse to listen to the message any longer).

Consider the catchy refrain from "Tea for Two" in the musical comedy *No, No, Nanette*, ". . . a boy for you, a girl for me. . . ." If this were the sole message women heard, they would (under our assumptions) produce families with an average of three children. This is not ZPG. Of course, not many of the world's 3.6 billion people have ever attended a performance of *No, No, Nanette*. But hundreds of millions of them have been exposed to the messages of Planned Parenthood. Multitudes of the illiterate people of the world have seen P-P billboards showing a happy mother and father with just two children—a boy and a girl. The message is unfortunately ambiguous. "Just two," is fine; but "a boy for you, a girl for me" is not. Which of these two messages comes across to poor and illiterate women? If the latter, as I suspect, they will not stop until they have produced three children (on the average), which is ruinous on a spaceship.

In India, the leading indigenous message is "an heir and a spare." For a complex of social reasons an Indian woman will be uneasy until she has at least two sons. Two sons means, on the average, four children. The result: a doubling of the population every generation. This is approximately what is happening in India. Her growth rate is 2.5 percent per year, yielding a doubling time of only twenty-eight years. Ruin comes on like a hurricane, and dignity goes out the window.

Birth control is not population control: perfect birth control merely permits women to have the number of children they want. There will be population control only if women want the right number of children. In every country in the world in which an attitude survey has been made with respect to family size, women want too many children to produce ZPG. Population growth will be achieved only when women's attitudes are changed; changing these is the goal of the second phase in population control.

2. Educational Phase

How do we change people's attitudes? By education, we say—but the word "education" hides a world of complexity. To be effective, education has to be tied to the culture; that means that education must vary from country to country, and from culture to culture. Let us restrict the discussion to the United States, which will supply us with quite enough difficulties.

We must give careful attention to the messages young children hear, particularly young girls, for these messages powerfully form their attitudes toward marriage and the family in later years. Some of the messages children are subjected to in our elementary schools encourage recklessness on board the spaceship.

Recall the Dick-and-Jane books. What is their population message? Simply this: *there is only one normal way to live*—HAVE CHILDREN. Dick and Jane's parents have children, of course; but so also do the neighbors on the left, those on the right, the ones across the street—in fact, all God's chillun have chillun. In the literal sense, anything else is *unthinkable*. Exposed at a tender age to such a message, what is a little girl to conclude? Plainly that she just has to become a mommy when she grows up. Nothing else is normal. That's the message of the Dick-and-Jane books.

I think it's time to change the message. We shouldn't get rid of it entirely; but we should augment it with another message, a contradictory one. Let us introduce first-graders to delightful Aunt Debbie—thirty years old, pretty as a picture, and fond of

Table 1. A SYSTEMS ANALYSIS OF POPULATION GROWTH DEMONSTRATING THAT BIRTH CONTROL IS NOT SYNONYMOUS WITH POPULATION CONTROL

Message	Reception	Performance	Fertility	Increase	Consequence
Society's Directives, Implicit or Explicit	Precision Assumed	Effectiveness of Birth Control Assumed	Approximate Average Number of Children per Family	Factor of Increase per Generation	Long-run Effects, in a Spaceship
"One's enough"	Perfect	Perfect	1	0.5	Depopulation; then extinction
"I must have an heir"	Perfect	Perfect	2	1 (ZPG)	Dignity possible
"Stop at two"	Perfect	Perfect	2	1 (ZPG)	Dignity possible
"A boy for you, a girl for me"	Perfect	Perfect	3	1.5	Ruin
"An heir and a spare"	Perfect	Perfect	4	2	Ruin
"Cheaper by the dozen"	Perfect	Perfect	12	6	Ruin

children (but only in small doses). She is a working woman and likes her job. She likes her freedom. She also likes men. The children just love her and look forward to her visits.

Jane, in the depths of her subconscious, wonders whether she wants to be like Mommy when she grows up, or like Aunt Debbie. She doesn't know. She just doesn't know.

And she shouldn't, not at her age. Let Jane grow up hearing two messages: being a mommy is nice—but so also is being a Debbie. Let her find her own identity. Later. And let society make it possible for her to live a psychologically rich and respected life if she decides that parenthood is not for her. We will all benefit if women are freed to find their own identities and not pressured into having children they do not want.

In the elementary grades we must keep the option of childlessness alive in the child's mind. At the secondary level we need to display a wide spectrum of enticing vocations available to nonparents. A significant part of our success in population control will come as a "fallout" from making it possible for more women to become scientists, artists, machinists, businesswomen—the list is endless. It even includes work in the nursery—the community nursery, that is—as professionals in child care. We not only have too many children, we have too many poorly taken care of. We need to pay women to fulfill this role, so important to the nation, instead of expecting them to be unpaid slaves. Paradoxical as it may seem, if we pay them well for taking care of children, they will probably breed less.

3. Coercive Phase

Some think this phase will never be needed. They may be right—but I think not, for the purely Darwinian reason that *voluntary population control selects for its own failure.* Noncooperators outbreed cooperators. It is inconceivable that a nation of hundreds of millions could be without its noncooperators, so we had better begin to think about a third phase of population control, a coercive phase.

I said *think about*—no more. Not yet. The dangers of coercion are grave. We would not run such dangers, ever, except that we live on a spaceship and know that purely voluntary population control is self-defeating. We must do a great deal of thinking about ways to keep coercion under control before we can safely act decisively.

We need imaginative social engineering. We can see farther than we can act.

Coercion is a spectrum, ranging from tax incentives to detention camps. Even government-financed persuasion—education—can be considered a form of coercion. It is tempting to opt for tax incentives as being a gentler form of coercion, one that is compatible with conventional ideas of freedom; but even these have dangers. If we tax parents for having too many children, some of the punishment is passed from the parents to the children, who are not, in any sense, responsible for the sins of their parents.

It has been suggested that the amount of a person's retirement annuity be inversely related to the number of children he or she has produced. This scheme would not harm the children, who should be on their own by the time their parents retire. There are, however, two substantial criticisms to be made of the proposal. First, it may be questioned whether the bait would in fact be effective. How many people, at the fertile age of twenty-five or thirty, believe *in their bones* that they will someday be old? How many will sacrifice the present pleasure (whatever it is) of having children for a problematical future pleasure of more money to spend in their dotage when (they rightly suspect) the edge of all pleasure is dulled? Besides, they may not live that long. (True.) Or the social system may collapse, wiping out their retirement fund. (This also is true, but it cannot even be discussed, without prejudice, by the Establishment that proposes a delayed reward for nonproductivity.)

The second objection to the proposal is more fundamental: this is but one more system that selects for its own failure. Those adults who respond to the incentive, and are rewarded, have fewer children than those who ignore it. If the difference between the two groups of parents depends on temperamental characteristics that are even in the slightest degree hereditary—foolhardiness? courage? prudence? philoprogenitiveness?—then the relative frequency of the genes that make for the desired response to the incentive will decrease with the succession of generations. It is hard to be enthusiastic about a scheme that is deficient on this most fundamental of grounds.

The economist Kenneth Boulding has proposed what he calls his "green stamp plan" to lower the birth rate by using the market mechanism long employed to allocate scarce material resources.

I have only one positive suggestion to make, a proposal which now seems so farfetched that I find it creates only amusement when I propose it. I think in all seriousness, however, that a system of marketable licenses to have children is the only one which will combine the minimum of social control necessary to the solution to this problem with a maximum of individual liberty and ethical choice. Each girl on approaching maturity would be presented with a certificate which will entitle its owner to have, say, 2.2 children, or whatever number would ensure a reproductive rate of one. The unit of these certificates might be the "deci-child," and accumulation of ten of these units by purchase, inheritance, or gift would permit a woman in maturity to have one legal child. We would then set up a market in these units in which the rich and the philoprogenitive would purchase them from the poor, the nuns, the maiden aunts, and so on. The men perhaps could be left out of these arrangements, as it is only the fertility of women which is strictly relevant to population control. However, it may be found socially desirable to have them in the plan, in which case all children both male and female would receive, say, eleven or twelve deci-child certificates at birth or at maturity, and a woman could then accumulate these through marriage.

This plan would have the additional advantage of developing a long-run tendency toward equality in income, for the rich would have many children and become poor and the poor would have few children and become rich. The price of the certificate would of course reflect the general desire in a society to have children. Where the desire is very high the price would be bid up; where it was low the price would also be low. Perhaps the ideal situation would be found when the price was naturally zero, in which case those who wanted children would have them without extra cost. If the price were very high the system would probably have to be supplemented by some sort of grants to enable the deserving but impecunious to have children, while cutting off the desires of less deserving through taxation. The sheer unfamiliarity of a scheme of this kind makes it seem absurd at the moment. The fact that it seems absurd, however, is merely a reflection of the total unwillingness of mankind to face up to what is perhaps its most serious long-run problem.

The general effect would be to allocate child-permits as we now allocate Cadillacs—to the richest. The scheme would fail to do this to the degree that there is a "philoprogenitive instinct," inheritable in the most general sense; to this degree the scheme would select for its own failure. But the scheme might be a useful interim measure in getting people used to the idea of parenthood as a licenseable privilege instead of a right.

We make people take driving tests before allowing them to drive cars, but any idiot can become a parent, which is an immensely more demanding activity.

There is only one way to eliminate the counterproductive effect of choice in population control, and that is to get rid of the choice itself. The logic of choice-exclusion is not new, merely the application of it to parenthood. We *might* allow freedom of choice in the robbing of banks; but we don't, because freedom of choice would favor robbers and select against conscience. Freedom would be counterproductive, with respect to widely accepted goals of society that we treasure even more than freedom. It is hardly necessary to spell these out.

Freedom to breed is also counterproductive in the same sense, but with this difference: it is only counterproductive beyond a certain level of population or population-growth rate. The morality of breeding is situation-sensitive. If we want to be equitable in the allocation of the right to breed, we must say that an individual has such a right until she has *n* children, but not beyond. Beyond *n* she has broken the law.

Laws that take account of situations present serious problems of enforcement. An absolute proscription is comparatively easy to enforce because it facilitates the linkage of emotion to law. Emotional reactions legitimate law. When a bank robber is caught, we are unhesitatingly against him. But what is our reaction to a killer of bears, if anyone with a license is allowed one bear per season? Before we know how to react to the killer, we have to know whether he has a license, what sort of gun he used, and whether this is in fact his first kill of the year. Such nit-picking tends to drain emotion from our reaction and endangers the legitimation of the law. This is one of the reasons why poaching is harder to control than murder.

Coercive control of population will be difficult. Even if we avoid the administrative rulings as to the limits, writing all limits into law, we still will need bureaus to ferret out the facts. This is unfortunate, doubly so at the present time because of the low esteem in which bureaus are held. "Bureaucratic" is a pejorative, almost solely so. But population control will never work without good bureaucratic implementation. This is one more reason why we will not soon achieve population control. In the meantime, pollution and the ills of overcrowding will get worse. We will have to stew in our own juices for a while longer.

As always in our society, worshipers of Progress have hoped that a technological "breakthrough" might relieve us of the necessity of making hard decisions in the ethical, social, and political realms. They have dreamed of a contraceptive that could be added to the water, thus making everyone automatically and safely sterile. The hypothetical contraceptive could be countered with an antidote available only on prescription from the population-control bureau. In the reverse of the present situation, sterility would be easy and automatic, fertility difficult.

The dream is seductive, but it does not really bypass the ethical, social, and political problems. We would still have to get community agreement to use the sterilizing agent.

In addition, the proposal is even technologically suspect. The chemist Carl Djerassi, one of the principals in the "pill" technology, has given a more than sufficient number of reasons for believing that a drinking-water contraceptive will never be found.

The pharmacological standards for an acceptable agent are extremely severe. It would have to be effective and not harmful over an extremely wide range of water intake. It would have to be stable in solution in contact with all the substances that make up pipes, valves, and water containers. It should have no adverse effects on children and old people, who don't need it. It should have no detectable side effects.

How would one control the problem of bootlegging untreated water? Or bootlegging antidotes?

How would one even *find* such a substance? The usual way of looking for a new substance is by *animal tests first,* then human tests. But the ideal substance would be one that sterilized humans only, and not our cats, dogs, horses, cows, and other domestic animals. Of course we might settle for less than the ideal, but in testing substances there would always be a chance that the perfect substance, as determined by animal tests, would be ineffective in humans. Contrariwise, a poor substance (according to animal tests) *might* be perfect for humans—but how would we ever find that out, following the "animals first" rule for testing new drugs?

Not in new technology will the answer be found to population control, but in new approaches to social and political change. We have no proven techniques for converting from one set of ethical standards to another—not painlessly.

How can the transition from a voluntary to a coercive system be made? Must it be by an intermediate stage that combines legal freedom with *de facto* guilt assignment to parents who have more than two children? Older citizens who had their four or six children long before they were aware of the population problem do not take kindly to being lectured at by nulliparous young females from Zero Population Growth, Incorporated. Nor do younger parents who are still weighing the merits of population control like to be subjected to "jawbone responsibility," in the absence of genuinely operational responsibility.

"Guilt-pushing" is an old and honored tradition in liberal reform movements. Whether guilt feelings are less painful than legal restraint may at least be doubted. Whether the cultivation of guilt makes for a healthy society may also be doubted. But anyone reading the left-wing press (of which the *New York Review of Books* is an example of quality) is left with no doubt that many individuals in that segment of our society denoted by the term "intellectuals" are quite literally addicted to guilt. (Or is guilt-pushing merely the last and despairing bludgeon of the reformer when he becomes convinced that he is impotent if restricted to cleaner weapons?)

We could certainly benefit by finding a healthier way to effect the transition from the present voluntary system of family population control to the coercive system we must ultimately accept. Is there a better way?. . . Social inventors will please step forward!

Part IV

How to Die: Euthanasia

Modern medicine can save people from an untimely death; it can also forestall the time of death. The idea of being kept alive as a "vegetable" is anathema to some; others cling to life, resenting the thought of someone speeding them on their way. "Death with dignity" has become a sort of battle cry; yet at the other end of the spectrum are people who fight for life and compel their doctors to keep them alive as long as technically possible. The discussions about death and dying have led to college classes for the young, hospices for the old, as well as conferences for doctors to learn how to talk about the inevitable with their fading patients.

In Part 4 we have included essays on the death of children as well as the elderly; we have also included an essay on the "Living Will." The first selection is by Elisabeth Kübler-Ross, who can take most of the credit for making us better able to talk about death. In a question-and-answer format, she has covered most of the issues. Kübler-Ross's "good death" is a natural death, not induced, but not prolonged by artificial means. Marya Mannes gives some background to the euthanasia movement in this country as well as in England, and pleads the case of the elderly who are kept alive by artificial means. Mannes seems to argue for positive euthanasia (doing something to speed death) as well as for negative (doing nothing to prevent death).

The article from the Right to Life League also gives some background, and challenges the theory of "prolonging death." It argues, as do the two essays that follow, that it is not necessary to use heroic (extraordinary) means to save life, but that a doctor is committed to try to save life through ordinary and usual means. Both Frederic Grunberg and Richard McCormick agree that a retarded child who can still have meaningful relationships with other people should be saved. McCormick says that the good of the child should be considered, not its "usefulness."

We end with an article by David Dempsey discussing the "Living Wills." Such documents have no legal weight, but presumably they carry a good deal of persuasion. Dempsey wonders about the wisdom of making such a will when young and healthy, although provisions for yearly updating have been added to the documents by the Euthanasia Society. Dempsey also asks several questions, such as: Do people have a right to decide when to die?

18

Prolongation of Life

Elisabeth Kübler-Ross

Terminally ill patients pose many problems to us during the course of their illness; perhaps the greatest come during the very end of their suffering. There is a point of no return, no chance of ever getting up again or of resuming any form of functioning existence. The patient may exist this way for weeks or months. When are we serving him better by doing less? Who decides when life-prolonging measures should be stopped? Who decides what ordinary or extraordinary means are? Do we have a right to shorten a life, no matter how meaningless to us?

These are the questions that come up in every workshop, in every seminar, on the care of the dying patient. As Erich Fromm says: "I think there is no such thing as medical ethics. There are only universal human ethics applied to specific human situations." It is this humanistic conscience, referring to the philosophic or religious humanistic tradition, which has to be our guide in every difficult case. We always have to put ourselves into the situation of the patient *first*, then consider the family and the staff's needs, because all of these will play a role in our final decision.

We should also find a new definition for "euthanasia" since it is used for "good death" (*e.g.*, the patient's own natural death without prolonging his dying process unduly), and for mercy killing, which has nothing to do with the original intent of the word euthanasia. To me this is the difference between allowing someone to die his own death or killing him. I am naturally in favor of the former and opposed to the latter.

But real situations are not that simple. There are many borderline cases where we truly wonder whether we should keep a

From *On Death and Dying* (New York: Macmillan, 1974), pp. 74-87. Published in London by Tavistock Publications Ltd. Reprinted by permission of the publishers.

nasal tube or an I.V. going or whether we are only prolonging the terminal suffering by a few more weeks or months. The most beautiful hospital for the care of such patients is probably the St. Christopher Hospice in London, under the directorship of Dr. Cecily Saunders. Her patients, most of them with terminal cancer, are kept comfortable with adequate pain-relief; no mechanical means or machines are used in the Hospice; and neither food nor visitor restrictions are known for those patients. The questions so often raised in this country do not occur in the British Hospice, simply because they apply "the true art of medicine" to every patient. They surround them with love, faith, and excellent medical-emotional support, which allows the patient to live until he dies. The Rose Hawthorne Hospital in Fall River, Massachusetts is a similar though smaller facility.

Why do we try to keep patients alive with "horrible diets and treatments" when we know death is very near?

We very often keep "patients alive with horrible diets and treatments," because we hope that such treatment will bring about a remission and the patient will be able to live a fairly normal existence for another few months or years. If a patient is full of cancer, and we have a new chemotherapy available, we may be tempted to use this new treatment in the hope of making the patient more comfortable and to delay his death. It is also used in order to find out if a certain cancer responds to the new treatment, and if it does we may be able to use it on other patients later on in an earlier stage of their cancer. It is sometimes difficult to say whether or not the side effects and the added restrictions are more difficult and painful than the natural disease. It is sometimes questionable whether these treatments are really for the benefit of the patient or are used for our own needs and because of our own inability to accept the patient's death.

What are your views on euthanasia?

I am totally opposed to any kind of mercy killing, but I am in favor of allowing the patient to die his or her own death, without artificially prolonging the dying process.

Does society have the right to keep alive those who are designated by fate or God to die? Aren't we playing God? What are your feelings on this?

I don't think we should keep people artificially alive when they are no longer functioning human beings. This may be playing God, but I think it is a duty of every physician to keep somebody alive in a functioning condition. God may have given the physician the wisdom and the knowledge to do this. I'm very opposed to keeping people alive who are functioning purely as organ systems due to some equipment that is hooked up to them.

What about a patient who dies on you? When do you try to resuscitate?

If there is any chance for a meaningful life with some degree of functioning and at least the ability to express and receive expressions of human feelings, you should resuscitate by all means. If a cancer-ridden patient is dying on you I would not resuscitate.

Is it a patient's right to decide when to turn off the machines?

Yes, it should be the patient's privilege to decide when he is no longer willing to go along with a certain extension of life which to him may not only be meaningless, but also very costly.

Is euthanasia ever legal in the United States?

There are as yet no statutes legalizing euthanasia, but the trend is in that direction. It is important to differentiate between euthanasia as the word was used in the past, when it meant a good death, and as it is now used to designate mercy killing, which I personally cannot ever see as a good death. I am in favor of allowing patients to die their own natural deaths, without undue prolongation of the dying process and prolonged suffering, but I am not in favor of giving patients an overdose to "relieve them of their suffering."

Regarding President Truman's death—would you comment on the public's feeling that these people belong to the public and their lives should be prolonged (against their personal wishes) because of an "obligation" to the public to keep them alive?

It is tragic that people in such exposed positions often have to suffer more. It is inhuman and inexcusable when we prolong the dying process to such an extent as President Truman and Eleanor Roosevelt had to suffer. The doctors certainly do it in good faith, but it is not in the service of the patient.

What are your thoughts about keeping people alive with machines in hospitals when they are terminally ill or have only a very slim chance of getting better?

I think any patient who has a chance of getting better should get all the technical assistance that we have available. Patients who are beyond medical help and whose organs are kept functioning only with machines are not benefiting from this kind of management, and we should have the courage to learn when to call it quits.

If the patient is unable to decide whether extraordinary means to prolong life are to be used then who is responsible? What happens when family members cannot agree?

The patient should always have the first voice. If the patient is in a coma, or if he is not of legal age, the family's opinion is usually considered next. If the family cannot agree (and in the case of children, their parents should not be asked to make such a horrible decision), a treatment team should meet and make the decision as a group. Our ideal treatment team includes the physician who treats the patient, any specialist who has been in on the case, a member of the clergy, the nurses, the social worker, and a consulting psychiatrist. This team should understand the needs not only of the dying patient, but also of his family. In the case of children we ask each other if we would continue treatment if this were our child. If the unanimous opinion is against any use of extraordinary means, we then present this decision to the family. We do not ask them for an opinion, but simply state our decision, adding that it would require a strong veto on their part to make us decide otherwise. In a case when the child died, the family did not have feelings of guilt to add to grief, nor the thought, "Maybe if we had added another treatment, Susie would still be alive." They thus have the opportunity to blame us for the death of the child when they are in the stage of anguish and anger. With comatose patients, when the family cannot agree, we try to make a group decision, involving not only the professional team, but also members of the family.

Will you speak briefly about your attitude toward physicians who, by prolonging life by exclusively artificial means, refuse to allow patients to die?

These are the physicians who have been trained to cure, to treat, to prolong life, and who have never had any instruction on how to be a physician to terminally ill patients. They have been trained to regard dying patients as a failure. They themselves usually have unresolved fears of death and they feel uncomfortable when "a patient dies on them." It takes understanding, patience, and communication to make these physicians aware that they are not helping the patient, nor do they resolve their own internal conflicts by these procedures.

Is it possible, when a person reaches a point of acceptance that he is to die soon, that he can no longer accept the fact that he can mentally overcome his physical disease, to allow him to die and not extend his life just for the sake of keeping him alive? This is his wish, to be allowed to die. How does one overcome the fear of how one will behave and not lose one's dignity when terminally ill? Also, the fear of being a burden on everyone else?

Many patients have reached their stage of acceptance, have expressed the wish to be allowed to die, and have been able to keep their equanimity and their dignity to the very end. If the patient's needs are respected, if he has been truly loved, he will not be afraid of being a burden to everyone else.

What would you do and how would you respond to a friend who lived in terror of a crippling stroke and could not rest unless assured that he would be mercifully put out of his misery if he became too helpless physically or mentally to end his own life?

I would not promise him that I would put him out of his misery, because I would not be able to do that. I could only promise him that I would help him to live until he dies, in spite of his limitations.

How does one help people who are ashamed of living, who think they do not deserve to live, because they may be different in some way? Also—in view of the overpopulation problem—does one have the right to allow sick people to die by denying them medicine?

I think people who are ashamed to live because of a handicap, or because they are different in some way, need professional help. This world has enough room, and should have enough love to accept people who are different no matter in what way. Overpopulation should never be a reason for helping people to die by denying them medication or through any other means. If we did this, we would soon end up in another Nazi society.

How do you deal with a family who wants the life of a patient prolonged, but the patient would like to be allowed to die?

This happens many, many times. It means that the patient has reached the stage of acceptance, but the family is behind in the stages of dying, maybe in the stage of denial, anger, or bargaining. In these cases, you spend all your time and effort on the family and help them work through their unfinished business, so that they can allow the patient to die, to "let go."

Do you believe in prolonging death by giving I.V. feedings when a patient is already unconscious and in a coma?

I think it depends a great deal on the patient. I have seen many unconscious patients who were in comas and were given intravenous feedings, and who are now walking around, healthy, happy, and functioning. If a patient has been unconscious and in a deep coma for a long time, I think his brain waves must be checked repeatedly to see if he is still really alive, or only kept "alive" by a machine. In the latter case, I would naturally stop the intravenous feedings.

You referred to the ping-pong game of deciding where the patient may die—at home, as he wants, or in a hospital, which is a costly workshop for the medical profession, where his life can be extended through intravenous and other means. Should we the medical professionals extend the life of the vegetating person? Wouldn't it be merciful to let him die? President Truman's case is a good example of this.

Yes, I think there is still too much ambivalence in most of us, not only as to where a patient may die, but also as to where to keep some of our difficult patients. We should ask the patient if he would prefer to return home or if he would prefer to stay in the hospital, where the care may be a bit easier than at home, especially now when there is usually a lack of visiting nurses, physicians who make house calls, or people to take care of the night watch, etc. If the family gets enough assistance, I think most patients would prefer to die at home, and I would do everything humanly possible to fulfill this wish.

Do you let patients decide when they want to die, or do you keep on giving medications and helping them until the end?

I give them only as much medication as is necessary to keep

them comfortable. I will help them until they die, but when they refuse to have any further dialysis or any further surgery, which may prolong their lives by a few weeks or perhaps months, I understand their wishes.

What can one say to the elderly dying cancer patient in a nursing home who is obsessed with the desire to go home? We checked it out and it is impossible for her to be at home.

I think you have to level with her and tell her honestly why it is impossible for her to go home. This is a reality that she may have to learn to face. If the reasons are questionable you may be able to help her family overcome their fears or anxieties. With a little additional help, such as visiting nurses, you may be able to convince the family to take their mother home to die. They need enough back support and someone they can call if they are in trouble.

Many patients want to die at home, or are almost forced to do so because of finances and hospital admission policies. The patients' families may also wish this. Would you please comment on how health service professionals can help these patients and families, or even help them arrive at a decision?

I'm very much in favor of allowing patients to die at home. Not for financial reasons especially, but because patients usually wish to die in their own familiar environment rather than to have their life artificially prolonged in a hospital where they can be visited only on a limited basis. If you share with a family the advantages of the last final days or weeks at home, many family members will then decide about the possibility or feasibility of such an arrangement. We have to train more homemakers and we do need more visiting nurses and physicians who make house calls before this is possible for many patients.

If a patient is beyond medical help and wants to go home to die, isn't that the same as euthanasia?

It is the same as euthanasia only if you translate the word as "a good death." It is not mercy killing. It means simply allowing the patient to die with peace and dignity in his own familiar environment, and I am proud each time I can make this possible.

Do you think we will ever permit a person to die with dignity, rather than to use gadgets to prolong life?

I think in spite of all our unhappiness with these extraordinary means and life-prolonging procedures, the majority of the world population still dies without gadgets, and it will hopefully always be so.

In view of the pending legislation on euthanasia, what are your feelings on the subject?

I find it sad that we have to have laws about matters like this. I think that we should use our human judgment, and come to grips with our own fear of death. Then we could respect patients' needs, and listen to them, and would not have a problem such as this.

A young intelligent man with a "brilliant future" ahead of him suddenly finds himself a quadriplegic. Does this man have the option to decide if he is to go on living with only his brain functioning or should he be allowed to choose to die with dignity? (That means discontinue all life-saving measures and drugs.)

I think any young man who finds himself in this predicament needs all the help he can get, to show him ways and means of still functioning as a total human being. There are many people in our chronic patient hospitals, and in our VA hospitals, who are quadriplegics. If you visited some of these patients and saw what they are able to do, you would be surprised to see that they find meaning in their lives and are productive. As long as they have their brains, as long as they can still think, and use their eyes and their ears, and communicate, they should be given all the help possible to show them that life can still be meaningful and beautiful. I would take such patients to others who have gone through such a crisis, and have found ways and means of functioning. We should not discontinue life-saving measures as long as the patient's brain is functioning. This is my personal opinion.

Who should decide how long to maintain "support systems," the patient, the family, the physician, or society? Must each case be individualized, or are there valid generalized criteria? What factors are considered, the family needs, the quality of life, or the expense?

As long as the patient can express his needs, I think we should maintain a support system, because it means that the patient is still a functioning human being. If the patient is nonfunctioning and not communicating, the family, the physician, and the interdisciplinary team have to get together and make a joint decision. Each case should be discussed on an individual basis. I don't think we have valid generalized criteria, except for the definition of death, as outlined in Henry Beecher's *Harvard Report.*

Aren't we playing God when we don't allow patients to die and we use drugs on them to keep them alive?

A child who formerly would have died from poliomyelitis is now kept alive by giving him a prophylactic medication to prevent the illness; an old woman who formerly would have died of pneumonia is now kept alive with antibiotics. Is this playing God?

What do you say to a patient who seriously requests mercy killing from the medical staff?

I have to find out first why he cannot bear his present situation anymore. Maybe he has so much pain that he can't tolerate it; then I have to increase his pain medication. If he has been deserted by his family, I see if I can contact the family. If he is a man who needs to be in control of his life and who cannot tolerate having no control over his dying, then I give him assistance so that he can control certain procedures, maybe the choice of his food, maybe the time of his bath, or the number of visitors he can have at the hospital. He then has the feeling that he is still in control of many things. If he signs himself out of the hospital and refuses to take medication, he has the right to do so. If the patient is not mentally ill, we have to allow him this decision. If he is mentally ill, I would naturally request a psychiatric consultation, and see if we can get him into a better emotional state to make this decision rationally and in accordance with his real wishes.

When a patient has reached acceptance and the family has accepted it too, why not remove the machinery that keeps the patient "alive"? If the hospital still wants to prolong the life, what can the family do to let the patient die with dignity?

A patient's family can always ask for a consultation. They can transfer the patient to another facility, or take him home. The simplest way, perhaps, but not always a successful one, is to talk to the physician in charge, to see if he can accept the decision reached by the patient and the family.

I do not favor euthanasia in reference to incurable diseases. But at what point should physicians decide to cease prolongation of life by life-saving methods and medication? I am thinking of the financial burden inevitably placed on the family left behind; sometimes it is overwhelming.

We found some very general rules, which we use often as guidelines in making these decisions. When the patient has reached the stage of acceptance and the family is also at peace, the patient often asks to stop all life-prolonging procedures. We would respect this request under most circumstances, especially if we are sure that the patient has no chance of cure or of a remission. This naturally does not mean that we discontinue the necessary fluid intake, and that we do not give them the necessary physical care and pain medication, if these are indicated. We would also at this time discuss the possibility of a transfer home with the family, in order to allow the patient to die in a familiar environment. If the family is taught how to give injections, if we notify the visiting nurses association, and if we as physicians make occasional house calls, most families are able to handle such patients quite well.

19

The Good Death

Marya Mannes

Euthanasia is a word that conjures up—still, in many people—almost as much fear as death itself. It is one thing to translate the Greek word into "the good death"; it is another to clear away the confusions about what, exactly, this apparently benign term means.

Is it something you do to yourself: suicide? Is it something others do to you: murder? Could it even be a polite synonym for genocide: mass killing of the innocent, young or old, who happen to be burdens on society?

—Euthanasia is none of these things. It is simply to be able to die with dignity at a moment when life is devoid of it. It is a purely voluntary choice, both on the part of the owner of this life and on the part of the doctor who knows that this is no longer a life.

Euthanasia is the chosen alternative to the prolongation of a steadily waning mind and spirit by machines that withhold death or to an existence that mocks life.

For the doctor, it is the passive or negative act of refraining from measures that in his opinion would sustain merely a marginal or vegetable existence. That he would be influenced by the express wish of a conscious patient to "let go" seems reasonable, though the decision is, and must be, primarily his own.

Suicide, whether approved by others or not, is the most solitary human choice. The definition of it as rational or irrational is entirely arbitrary.

As for mercy killings, they are dual acts. One human being helps another to end intolerable suffering; sometimes on the single

From *Last Rights* (New York: William Morrow and Co., Inc., and London: Millington House, 1974), pp. 60-72, 80-86. Copyright © 1973 by Marya Mannes. Reprinted by permission of the publishers.

initiative of compassion and horror, more often in response to the pleas of the sufferer. Mercy is not strained.

And abortion? Here the choice is complex, involving mother, doctor, and unborn fetus. In the case of a fetus found to be so severely damaged in brain or body or both that its birth would mean merely a vegetable life, the termination of this life could indeed be called "the good death." The only difference between the vegetable old and the vegetable young is the length of time inexorably facing the child and its stricken parents.

We are in many ways a violent society, reacting violently to various forms of oppression, real or presumed, by official fiat or human prejudice. But a nation in which capital punishment even for major crimes is increasingly rare would find it hard to justify the killing of its political or social rejects in the name of euthanasia.

We would do better as citizens to exchange such apocalyptic fears of possible ultimate evil for the increasing realities of a possible ultimate good.

The idea of euthanasia has been a long time coming.

In all societies, the structure of power of state or church has consistently rejected any idea likely to give the individual power of choice in matters of life and death, or freedom of action in accord with his own private conscience. The only way any ruling establishment until recent times has been able to maintain its sovereignty, in fact, has been able to keep people within frameworks of legal and religious patterns which may once have served society well, but have now—in the light of mighty convulsions—ceased to be either applicable or useful in human terms.

Yet single courageous voices have never been stilled. In 1624, John Donne, the Dean of St. Paul's, wrote an essay in support of euthanasia asking ["whether it was logical to conscript a young man and subject him to risk of torture and mutilation in war and probable death, and refuse an old man escape from an agonizing end."]

Even earlier Sir Thomas More, eminent Catholic, wrote in the second book of his *Utopia* that in his imaginary community "when any is taken with a torturing and lingering pain, so that there is no hope either of cure or ease, the priests and magistrates come and exhort them, that, since they are not able to go on with the business of life, are becoming a burden to themselves and all about them, and they have really outlived themselves, they should no longer nourish such a rooted distemper, but choose rather to die since they cannot live but in much misery."

And in his *New Atlantis,* Francis Bacon wrote: "I esteem it the office of a physician not only to restore health, but to mitigate pain and dolours; and not only when such mitigation may conduce to recovery, but when it may serve to make a fair and easy passage."

"A fair and easy passage." Less than a century ago, anesthetics to ease the passage of birth or the pain of an operation were considered offenses against "God's will" by the pious.

In 1847, an Edinburgh physician gave ether to women in labor, a year after Massachusetts General Hospital in Boston began using it in surgery. He was attacked by the profession, laity, and clergy, who claimed that the pains of labor were appointed to the lot of women by divine decree, and that it was sacrilegious to use means for their relief.

"It is a decoy of Satan," intoned a minister of the Gospel, "apparently offering itself to bless woman, but in the end will harden society and rob God of the deep, earnest cries for help which arise in time of trouble." The good minister, of course, had never given birth. Neither have legislators opposing abortion, nor, since they are clearly not at death's door, those opposing euthanasia.

Church and state are simply continuing the kind of attacks made in turn by their supporters against vaccination, the ligation of arteries, the telescope, and the microscope. Anything, in fact, that might alter the prevailing attitudes toward the meaning of life or death, or extend human perception.

And yet long before Christ, Greek mythology encouraged Greeks suffering from incurable ailments to entreat Thanatos, the god of death, to free them from their misery.

And long after Christ, in our first years as a nation, Benjamin Franklin, referring to man's painful end, said, "We have very great pity for an animal if we see it in agonies and death throes. We put it out of its misery no matter how noble the animal."

Basically, the core of this unending argument is the contradiction implicit in the Hippocratic Oath, which promises two things: first, to relieve suffering, and second, to prolong and protect life. Yet often the prolongation of life can increase pain; and the relief of pain can shorten life.

Since the Hippocratic Oath was defined in 400 B.C. and in

increasing numbers of medical colleges is no longer required, many doctors might turn gratefully to the law to help them resolve this acute dilemma of conscience. But attempts to enact legislation permitting voluntary euthanasia within strict and clearly defined limits and conditions have been struck down in Great Britain successively in parliamentary debates of 1936, 1950, and 1969, and in the New York State Legislature in 1947. This particular bill was underwritten by almost two thousand physicians and fifty-four clergy, the latter denounced by the 1947 American Council of Christian Churches as "evidence that the modernistic clergy have made further departure from the eternal moral law."

Since the unsuccessful New York State bill of 1947 was a simpler version of the first British attempt to introduce legal euthanasia, it might be illuminating to give the essence of the last debate in the House of Lords in 1969 on the "good death."

(It is wryly typical of British mores that Lord Raglan's powerful arguments for euthanasia were preceded by an amendment offered by a Lord Hughes that "will have the effect of repealing completely the present order authorising the use of gin traps against both foxes and otters. The order will not be repealed only in so far as it applies to otters, which I am sure was the intention of the noble Lord, Lord Burton.")

After mentioning the previous efforts to legalize euthanasia, Lord Raglan said:

"I think that I have good reason to believe that opinion generally has become so favourable to a change in the law that the time is ripe, not to bring a Motion to test your Lordships' opinion but to introduce another Bill incorporating changes in the proposed formalities and safeguards, which I think were rightly criticised in the previous Bill, and which I, with some confidence, hope your Lordships will think a sound basis for legislation. When my noble friend Lord Langford was criticising the Abortion Bill he made a prophecy that it would be 'euthanasia next.' In fact, it was quite a safe prophecy to make, because this Bill, as I see it, is one in line with recent measures, such as the Suicide Act and others, which betoken a change of attitude in our society towards the freedom of the individual."

Raglan went on to observe that there was now less inclination for the state to legislate in areas of private conscience and behavior than before, and that in fact there was growing demand for repeal or modification of existing laws that seemed unduly restrictive of private choice.

He found it surprising that voluntary euthanasia had not already become legal, and believed the main reason for this was that those who most wished for it—the old and infirm—could not of necessity wage an energetic and articulate campaign.

"Those who suffer and die slowly," said Raglan, "may not have much to say for themselves; and death itself is the most private experience of all."

This introductory statement was followed by eight major clauses:

Clause 1 provides that a physician may administer euthanasia to a "qualified patient" who has made a declaration in the form set out in the schedule. A qualified patient is defined as a patient over the age of majority who has been certified by two physicians, one being of consultant status, to be apparently suffering from an irremediable condition.

Clause 2 provides that a declaration shall come into force thirty days after being made, and shall remain in force for three years. A declaration reexecuted within the twelve months preceding its expiry date shall remain in force for life, unless revoked.

Clause 3 provides that a declaration may be revoked at any time.

Clause 4 provides that before euthanasia may be given to a mentally responsible patient the physician in charge must ascertain to the best of his ability that the declaration and steps proposed to be taken under it accord with the patient's wishes. Subsection (2) provides that a nurse, acting on the directions of a physician, may cause euthanasia to be administered to a patient, and subsection (3) provides that no physician or nurse who is opposed on principle to euthanasia shall be required to take any steps in its administration.

Clause 5 protects physicians and nurses who act in good faith in the belief that their actions are in accordance with a patient's declaration or further requests made under the Act and provides that they *shall not be in breach of any professional oath by administering euthanasia.*

Clause 6 provides that a person who conceals, destroys, falsifies, or forges a declaration commits an offense punishable by life imprisonment and that an attesting witness who willfully makes a false statement commits an offense punishable by up to seven years' imprisonment.

Clause 7 provides that euthanasia shall not, except in limited circumstances, invalidate any insurance policy.

Clause 8 declares that all terminal patients are entitled to receive whatever quantity of drugs may be required to keep them entirely free from pain; and that in a case where severe distress cannot be alleviated by pain-killing drugs, the patient is entitled, if he so desires, to be made and kept entirely unconscious. The section applies to patients whether or not they have made any declaration, and is expressed to be for the removal of doubt as to the existing state of the law.

The clauses were followed in turn by a detailed definition of all terms involved, including "physician," "qualified patient," "irremediable condition," and so forth.

Although Raglan's bill was supported by a substantial minority, some criticized it as being too cumbersome or restrictive both for lawyers and doctors, believing that a simplified version would attain its ends without such complex means.

Others continued to view any efforts to legalize euthanasia, however guarded, as the "thin edge of the wedge."

Simply, it means that any departure from, or intrusion of, the statutes of common law that we inherited from the British and incorporated into our own Constitution, is a violation of basic ethics and an invitation to evil. In the context of euthanasia, "mercy killing" of the dying becomes simply murder, and suicide, self-murder.

The religious objection is, of course, founded on the Sixth Commandment, commonly translated as "Thou shalt not kill," but actually phrased in the Book of Common Prayer as "Thou shalt do no murder."

In both cases it is assumed that any act terminating a life from motives of mercy or compassion can—if permitted by law—be inspired as well by evil motives.

We come here to a curious anomaly. Mass killing as in war is not included in these pulpit strictures against "murder." Since supreme domination over life belongs to God alone, God alone may authorize man to kill, although in the words of the Reverend Joseph V. Sullivan, "today there is no indication that God is giving anyone orders to kill the innocent."

"Innocent" apparently does not apply to a combatant opposing a nation "that is fighting a just war, or an unjust aggressor."

This might explain the ardor with which two eminent American churchmen, the late Cardinal Spellman, and his successor Cardinal Cooke, supported our war in Vietnam while saying prayers for thousands of American dead. No prayers were said for the several million "unjust aggressors" killed by Americans.

This continuing paradox of the "wedge" principle (the assumption that every new concept, however benevolent in purpose, can also serve malign ends) would make it impossible to draw the line, because the line would have to be pushed further and further back until all action, for benign as well as evil motives, would be outlawed.

John Donne would have had no part of this: ". . . to chuse is to do: but to be no part of any body, that is to be nothing."

To be part of somebody is to feel for somebody. Some call this compassion, some empathy. If either is felt, benevolent action must proceed from it. It is hard to imagine that evil ends impel a doctor to remove the life supports of a dying patient. What malicious intent would prompt a physician to administer sedatives to ease terminal pain, knowing that nevertheless they might shorten the patient's life? The physician gains nothing from the death of a patient except a sense, perhaps, of defeat or—if the patient is a friend—of loss.

Cynics might suspect that some relatives might encourage the hastening of death not only because of the emotional and financial burdens of sustaining a flickering, helpless life, but for a hastened inheritance.

Yet even in such venal cases, feelings of guilt would probably deter action and be expiated by the greater burden of watching prolonged human deterioration. The doctor now hears, "Please don't do anything more" far oftener than he did ten years ago. And thousands of doctors now answer the plea.

My brother and I asked this of our family physician as the ninety-two-year-old father we loved so much was losing all substance except for his wish to die.

"Why must I go on?" he asked me one day. "Why?" And when I saw the stern Lutheran nurse who had replaced his former gentle companion try to force food into his mouth while he tried in vain to turn his face away, no doubts lingered. The doctor ordered the end of all artificial sustenance and chemical injections and our father was answered with death. This was, of course, one form of passive euthanasia: doing nothing to help sustain a guttering life. A life, in this case, bereft of joy, of will, of consciousness most of the time, and of the music which, along with a wife now ten years dead, were his imperative supports.

There are many variations of this "letting go." One doctor, knowing that one of his patients had no hope of survival, sent him home from the hospital on the grounds that he would be happier in familiar surroundings. Withdrawn from all artificial life supports, he died a week later, "quietly," said his wife, "in his sleep."

An elderly internist who treated an old friend of mine told me about G.'s last months. "As you know," he said, "G. had long been a diabetic, injecting himself daily with insulin before I treated him for leukemia. He was going on with his work, as well as he could, and coming to me every week for these new injections. In spite of them, of course, he grew progressively weaker until one day he turned up at my office, gray-faced, and said, 'Let me go. I am so tired. I don't want any more injections.'

"Because I not only loved but respected him greatly, I said, 'All right.' He died two weeks later, at home, in peace."

In both of these cases, the quality of life and not its extension was the overriding determinant. To certain individuals—usually those who have led full, demanding, and stimulating lives—the slow, inexorable reduction of their capacities is worse than death.

Possibly these are still a minority. Anyone in close contact with the long-term and critically ill will tell you that the will to live—consciously or unconsciously, and on whatever crippling or diminishing terms—is tenacious. The wards and nursing homes of this nation are full of half-lives, sustained by this tenacity.

The inference here might be that those who opt for life on any terms have never known life in its fullest terms. One of many alarming facts of our current society is the steady erosion of quality in the face of quantity. Too many people, surrounded by too many things, have too little. Not in terms of worldly goods but in the conscious savoring of the hours and days of their lives. Millions have never lived to their fullest capacities. And because of this, they would settle rather for a minimal life than no life at all. Their dread of death supersedes all else.

In sharp contrast are those human beings endowed since youth with a strong sense of purpose, of mission. For every genius in history who died young after fulfilling a creative destiny, there are a great number of individuals of marked attainments in the arts and sciences and government who, at whatever age, die soon after they can no longer function in their chosen work. They may have loving mates and children, but their impotence as productive beings is the paramount factor. In effect, they say, "My work is done." Their death is close to an act of will.

In the last twenty years we have seen this will thwarted by medical science, in the name of respect and even compassion, by keeping two Presidents half-alive far beyond their human needs or competence. The long-drawn-out ends of Eisenhower and Truman divested them both of the dignity of timely death. And although they were very different men, one could reasonably suspect that neither of them would have consciously chosen to die in the trap of machines and meaningless time.

Among humbler mortals, the element of will or choice takes another form. Especially in devoted and long-married couples, the death of the one is followed often and usually soon by the death of the other. They cannot, literally, live without each other; and the death of the survivor seems neither accident nor coincidence. That this mysterious mechanism of will exists in many of us, consciously or subconsciously, deserves far more attention than it has so far been given.

I believe that the will to die is the direct reflection of the quality of life. And if that quality is indeed being debased by the mounting brutality, boredom, fragmentation, and frustration that mark our society, then the conscious choice in the very ill or severely maimed or old for a "good death," is a wholly valid one, to be honored by us all, including the doctors empowered to help them achieve it.

. . . . .

Mercy Killing

Once more, the interweaving of notes and phrases in this complex oratorio of death brings euthanasia and mercy killing together— echoes and conjunctions. Euthanasia concerns the desire of one person to cease living and the act of one doctor to permit death in circumstances of incurable suffering or terminal disease. Mercy killing is the conscious act of one person toward another, of any age, performed to spare the other from an intolerable life.

The classic mercy killing of our time occurred in the early fifties and was widely reported in the press far beyond the New England town where it happened. One account written by Dean Sperry of the Harvard Divinity School touched the salient points of the case:

A country doctor in New Hampshire, Dr. Herman N. Sander, was arrested on the charge of murder. He had had as a patient in the Hillsboro County Hospital a fifty-nine-year-old woman who was dying of cancer. She had wasted from 140 pounds to 80 pounds. The end was inevitable and very near. Torn with pity for her suffering he had given her in a vein four lethal injections of air, 10 cubic centimeters each. The frothy blood that resulted formed an embolus of which she died within ten minutes. He then entered on the hospital records an account of what he had done, and let the matter rest there.

The heads of the hospital, going over the case record of the patients at a staff meeting, came across this entry and reported it to the state. A warrant for the doctor's arrest was issued and served by the sheriff, charging that Dr. Sander "feloniously and willfully and of his own malice aforethought did inject. . . air into the veins of Abbie Borroto, and with said air injection, feloniously, willfully and of his said malice aforethought killed and murdered" his patient. The doctor pleaded not guilty, was released on $25,000 bail, and bound over for a hearing before the grand jury. Two days later, the grand jury remanded him for trial.

All reports indicated that Dr. Sander was a trusted and honored practitioner. His father had been an official of the Public Service Corporation of New Hampshire. As an undergraduate, he had captained the ski team at Dartmouth during his college days and had been a member of the college symphony orchestra. He had recently returned from a trip to Europe, where he had been studying socialized medicine, and was scheduled for a number of lectures on the subject. There was no question of any prior illegality in his practice, and his record was above reproach.

As for his act on this occasion, he said that he had done no wrong. The woman was within hours of her death. Prompted by pity, he had merely hastened what would have been the end in any case. On the Sunday after his arrest, he went with his family to the Congregational Church in Candia, as was his custom. His minister publicly expressed sympathy for him, while the minister of the First Congregational Church in the nearby city of Manchester preached a stirring sermon in his defense. The latter clergyman said that if the doctor was guilty, he too was guilty: for he had often prayed that some suffering parishioner might be "eased into the experience of death." Later in the day, 605 of the 650 registered voters in the town of Candia presented Dr. Sander with an unqualified testimonial as to his integrity and good name, telling him to use it hereafter as he might see fit.

Meanwhile, the attorney-general of New Hampshire, who was Dr. Sander's personal friend, said that "the case will be presented forcefully and in complete detail, regardless of personalities and theories involved, to the end that justice may be met." At the time of writing it was impossible to tell what the result of the ensuing trial would be.

The whole affair brought the arguments of mercy killing to a head. The Euthanasia Society of America had been agitating over some years for a change in the laws, to allow mercy killing. They suggested that such killing had been tacitly practiced by many physicians and that this irregular practice, which they held to be desirable and morally defensible, should be legally regularized. An officer of the society visited New Hampshire and said that they regarded this incident as a concrete example of the need for euthanasia. They hoped that the State of New Hampshire might, as a result, legalize mercy killing.

According to Dr. Sperry, the act of Dr. Sander conformed in theory to the program proposed by the Euthanasia Society. "Dr. Sander differed from the Society mainly in this, that he took the law into his own hands and went ahead on his own account. The nurse who had handed him the syringe that he used apparently had no knowledge of what he was doing and was cleared of any suspicion of being *particeps criminis*. Had he not duly entered the transaction on the hospital records he would probably have gone scot free. One can only conclude that, in making the entry after the act, he deliberately intended to make of his private act a public test case."

This Dr. Sander most certainly did. Had he not dictated notes for the case record to Miss Josephine Connor, the record librarian at the county hospital, and had Miss Connor not touched off the investigation, Sander would never been brought to trial.

And although hundreds of his fellow townspeople, his patients, and his colleagues offered to testify on his behalf and signed petitions urging the courts to dismiss his case, a grand jury indicted him for first-degree murder. "All that I can say," said Sander, "is that I am not guilty of any legal or moral wrong and ultimately my position will be vindicated."

It was; and not long afterward he was acquitted. Although his license to practice was temporarily suspended and certain pastors fulminated against him from their pulpits—among them the Reverend Billy Graham, who said in Boston that "Dr. Sander should be punished as an example" and that "anyone who voluntarily, knowingly or premeditatedly takes the life of another, even one minute prior to death, is a killer"—most public sentiment was for him. (So have most juries, presented with similar cases, rendered "not guilty" verdicts.)

After he had supported himself and his family for a period as a farmhand for four dollars an hour, the Medical Board of the State of New Hampshire eventually reinstated his license, and he has since spent peaceful years of practice in his home town.

Even so, and even now, there is nowhere in the common law any toleration for mercy killing. The condemning thunder of Blackstone, deity-father of common law and hence of the body of most of our inherited statutes, rolls on, whether euthanasia, abortion, suicide, or mercy killing is in question.

Speaking of accessories to suicide, he observes: "The law in such cases can only reach the man's reputation and fortune. Hence, it has ordered an ignominious burial in the highway with a stake driven through the offender's body and the forfeiture of his goods and chattels to the king."

Thus, through the wisdom and mercy of God, was the sanctity of life sustained—in the eyes of the righteous.

In the eyes of the just, on the other hand, one would be more inclined to echo the words of one Roman citizen reacting to a famous mercy killing some years ago in his city. "It would have to happen to you before you could know what to do."

This concerned a young father who dropped his deformed infant son from a bridge to his death in the Tiber River.

The baby, Ivano, was born without legs or fingers. The twenty-nine-year-old father, Livio Davani, was in jail on a charge of murder. The minimum penalty was ten years in prison.

"My son would never have forgiven me if I had let him live only to suffer," Davani told police when he gave himself up.

Out of one hundred Romans interviewed by the capital's independent newspaper, *Il Messaggero,* twenty-two said they would have done what the father did; thirty-one said they would not; forty-seven did not know.

Davani, a photoengraver, had gone to San Camillo Hospital and taken out his son, born twenty-eight days earlier. For four hours he drove through the streets. Then he stopped his car and carried the baby halfway across the Flaminian Bridge.

" 'I took off his little dress,' the father was quoted as saying, 'and saw again how he was deformed. He began crying, because it was time for his bottle. I could no longer resist. Grown, he would have cursed me. I don't care how long they keep me in prison. Now I am more serene.'

"His wife, Nada, who talked with him half an hour in jail, said she would appeal to President Giuseppe Saragat for clemency. 'He is not an assassin,' she said. 'He did it for the baby. He could not let it suffer.' Prosecutor Mario Schiavotti, charging Davani with willful homicide, said, 'It's tragic but that's the law. What can I do?' "

The defense attorney, one of Italy's leading criminal lawyers, planned to contend that Davani acted under irrestible emotional strain, and the Vatican newspaper *L'Osservatore Romano* commented that "evidently the father was the victim of psychological shock which demands tremendous compassion." But it added: "Human life is a gift of which God is the supreme judge and of which only He can dispose."

Would the Vatican writer have wanted to live his life without legs or fingers? It would seem that strict adherence to faith can at one and the same time provide personal solace, yet also a shield against that empathy which permits one to suffer what others suffer and understand why they do what they must do.

The quality of mercy cannot be strained when mercy inspires the act under judgment. And when the law and the Church can find no distinction between good and evil intent, they have abdicated their service to humanity.

Now, here in America, this distinction has become vital, whether the object of "mercy killing" or active euthanasia is a deformed and mindless infant or the human wreckage of a car crash, multiple fractures and concussion leading to irreversible coma. Whether the one who ends this half-life is a doctor or a parent or a loving friend, the inherent mercy of such an act should weigh heavily in its favor where legal or moral judgment is concerned.

Since God cannot dispose of these "gifts of life" which have turned to curses, then man will have to.

20

Voluntary Euthanasia: The Right to Be Killed

Frank J. Ayd, Jr.

Does a man suffering with severe, intractable pain due to an incurable illness and whose death is inevitable and imminent have the moral right to have voluntary euthanasia? Yes, say euthanasiasts. And, since he has the moral right to be killed, he should have the legal right. Hence, in the past three decades in England and in the United States organized Euthanasia Societies have been working diligently to have voluntary euthanasia legalized.

Proposals Put Forward in the Past

In 1935, the Euthanasia Society in England was founded. The next year a bill was introduced in the House of Lords which sought to permit voluntary euthanasia in certain circumstances, and with certain safeguards. This bill provided:

> That the patient should first sign an official Form of Application stating his wish to anticipate death by euthanasia, and declaring that he had consulted his nearest relative about that decision. There had to be two witnesses to his signature, one of them a magistrate, or a solicitor, or a doctor, or a clergyman. The application should be forwarded within seven days to a "euthanasia referee appointed under the Act," together with certificates by two medical men as to the fatal character of the patient's illness and the degree of his suffering. The Minister of Health should then arrange for one or more referees to visit the patient and satisfy himself that the latter had understood his request, and that his condition was as specified by the doctors. The permission for euthanasia should not take effect for three days after being

Reprinted by permission of the author. This was first published in *The Medical-Moral Newsletter*, January-February 1970.

granted by the referee. In the meantime the patient's nearest relative should be informed and he could, if he so wished, apply to a Court of Summary Jurisdiction which could suspend the permit if there was reason to doubt whether all the conditions had been complied with.

During the discussion of this bill, Lord Dawson of Penn remarked: "This is a courageous age, but it has a different sense of values from the ages which have gone before. It looks upon life more from the point of view of quality than of quantity. It places less value on life when its usefulness has come to an end. There has gradually crept into medical opinion, as it has crept into lay opinion, the feeling that one should make the act of dying more gentle; and also more peaceful, even if it does involve curtailment of the length of life." Despite many speeches urging passage of this bill, after its second reading it was rejected by 35 votes to 14.

During the late 1930s in the United States, Dr. Charlotte Gilman, while dying of cancer, wrote: "When all usefulness is over, when one is assured of an imminent and unavoidable death, it is the simplest of human rights to choose a quick and easy death in place of a slow and horrible one. Public opinion is changing on this subject. The time is approaching when we shall consider it abhorrent to our civilization to allow a human being to lie in prolonged agony which we should mercifully end in any other creature. Believing this choice to be of social service in promoting wider views on this question I have preferred chloroform to cancer."

Responsive to such views the Euthanasia Society of America was formed. Immediately it began to push for the legalization of voluntary euthanasia. In 1947, a bill was put before the New York State General Assembly. It provided for the following:

1. Any sane person over twenty-one years old, suffering from an incurably painful and fatal disease, may petition a court of record for euthanasia, in a signed and attested document, with an affidavit from the attending physician that in his opinion the disease is incurable;

2. The court shall appoint a commission of three, of whom at least two shall be physicians, to investigate all aspects of the case and to report back to the courts whether the patient understands the purpose of his petition and comes under the provisions of the act;

3. Upon a favorable report by the commission the court shall grant the petition, and *if it is still wanted by the patient* euthanasia may be administered by a physician or any other person chosen by the patient or by the commission.

Although there were many who were sympathetic to the principle of voluntary euthanasia, they were opposed to this particular proposal because of the elaborate safeguards against abuse in it. This coupled with other arguments against voluntary euthanasia led to the defeat of this Bill.

In 1950, the House of Lords in England again debated another proposal for voluntary euthanasia essentially the same as the one debated in 1936. This proposal was withdrawn because of the opposition to it. The objections to the bills introduced in England and New York were varied. Some disliked the idea of the sick room being disturbed by so many legal formalities. Others feared the possible abandonment of the voluntary principle and the extension of permission to cover the case of mentally defective children or unwanted senile old people. Many felt that it was best to leave the matter for the time being to the discretion of individual physicians. They argued, correctly, that some deaths are almost certainly hastened by compassionate doctors with or without the consent, tacit or otherwise, of the sufferers.

Trends in Medical Opinion

Undaunted by their failures to have voluntary euthanasia legalized, the pro-euthanasiasts proceeded to cultivate what some of them call a "death-conditioned society." Their cause was aided considerably by the publication of two books strongly favoring euthanasia and by medical and technological advancements that enable physicians to prolong life, or as many aver, to prolong the act of dying. The former were written by an American Protestant theologian, Joseph Fletcher (*Morals and Medicine*), and by a prominent British attorney, Dr. Glanville Williams (*The Sanctity of Life and the Criminal Law*).

Physicians generally proclaim that all men have the right to die with dignity, just as they have a right to live with dignity. Yet there are divergent views on the doctor's duty when caring for a dying patient. Some contend that a doctor is required to do everything possible to preserve life. Many physicians argue that no one knows when death is inevitable. These men cite numerous instances of apparently hopeless cases snatched from the clutches of death and restored to a useful life for some years. That this is true is indisputable. Anyone acquainted with intensive care units in modern hospitals knows that many lives are saved daily by so-called heroic treatment. These successes amply justify the existence of these special units with their skilled physicians, nurses, and plethora of life-saving drugs and apparatus.

The apologists of intensive care units also point out that the knowledge gained from those who die in spite of vigorous efforts to save them may be applied successfully to future patients. What they have inherited from their predecessors enables them to use today's desperate and dramatic measures. They hope to will to their successors the fruits of their labor. They rightfully insist that what is extraordinary now will be ordinary in the future. Such is the tradition of progress in medicine.

An editorial captioned "Heroic Treatment" succinctly states the position of those who champion the use of all therapeutic measures to prolong life (*Medical Tribune,* April 10, 1961). Its author writes:

From time to time we are criticized for the overly dramatic and desperate treatment of moribund patients—for so surrounding the poor soul with infusions, oxygen, pressor amines, residents, and attendings that the relatives can barely have a glimpse of him amid a forest of equipment. The effort is sourly criticized as a "prolongation of death," not of life, and a plea is made for the dignity of a patient's last hours when he ought to be allowed to die in peace. [However] heroic treatment can succeed. As a result, quite a few "moribund" patients afterward stride out of the hospital in defiance of any reasonable judgment at the time of admission.

No one decries the laudable achievements in medical science from which brilliant life-saving measures derive. But for many years some doctors have criticized their colleagues for using heroic measures to prolong the act of dying. Almost two centuries ago Dr. J. Ferriar cautioned: "The Physician will not torment his patient with unavailing attempts to stimulate the dissolving system, from the idle vanity of prolonging the flutter of the pulse for a few more vibrations: if he cannot alleviate his situation, he will protect his patient against every suffering. . . . When things come to the last and the act of dissolution is imminent. . . he should be left undisturbed."

In an edifying lecture on "The Care of The Dying" in 1950, Dr. Alfred Worcester said:

> It is the physician's duty to protect the patient from the disturbance of officiousness: "Disturb him not, let him pass peaceably." Modern methods of resuscitation are most decidedly out of place where by disease or accident the body's usefulness has ended. Especially is this true where resuscitation would only renew the patient's sufferings. Such attempted defiance of nature is even less justifiable than are the efforts for prolonging life when the inevitable approach of death offers merciful release. Yet, in both of these ways, so many of our profession seem to believe themselves in duty bound to do their utmost. They ought to know better. The dying ought to be allowed to depart in peace.

With some justification an increasing number of doctors have voiced objections to "the obscenity of modern dying—a ritual sacrifice on the altar of technology" and to "the modern epidemic of resuscitation." Some have gone so far as to inform their physicians and relatives and to carry on their person a card stating "I do not wish to be resuscitated. I want to die with dignity—and for ever." These practitioners of the healing art agree wholeheartedly with Sir Theodore Fox, who said to his medical colleagues: "We shall have to learn to refrain from doing things merely because we know how to do them."

Doctors are not the only critics of modern medical ministrations to the dying. Lay people who have witnessed an expiring loved one's ordeal prolonged by oxygen, stimulants, and tubes inserted into natural and surgically created bodily orifices also have been censorious. They resent being deprived of the opportunity to share the waning moments of life with the one they love. For years they have shared joys and heartaches. Why, when they could face the greatest of all crises together, must they be shoved out of the room, displaced by gadgets and personnel striving to delay the inevitable? Some of those who have had such an experience have been constrained to voice their anguish and their hostility toward the medical profession.

An example of this feeling among the laity may be found in the January 1957 issue of the *Atlantic Monthly* which contains a poignant essay, entitled "A Way of Dying," by an anonymous authoress. This compassionate woman wrote:

There is a new way of dying today. It is the slow passage via modern medicine. If you are very ill modern medicine can save you. If you are going to die it can prevent you from so doing for a very long time. . . . We cannot inquire from the dead what they have felt about this deterrent. As they fight for spiritual release, and are constantly dragged back by modern medicine to try again, does their agony augment? To those who stand and watch, this seems like a ghastly imposition against God's Will be done—this incredible battle between spirit and medicine.

Euthanasia advocates have seized upon the growing opposition to the use of all therapeutic techniques to preserve life to urge those who feel this way to endorse voluntary euthanasia. They argue that it is even more compassionate for doctors to enable some individuals to escape from useless suffering, when, because of that suffering or a very serious disability, their continued existence no longer affords them pleasure or satisfaction. They are delighted with the views of physicians like Dr. Walter Alvarez who is not only opposed to prolonging a person's suffering, but also favors euthanasia. In a recent editorial (*Modern Medicine,* April 25, 1969) Dr. Alvarez wrote:

It will probably be many years before we [physicians] in America can bring ourselves to chloroform an idiotic infant or to permit a slowly dying patient to take an overdose of some sedative. Perhaps he is in great and constant pain and begging for an overdose of medicine. What we will first have to train ourselves to do will be to leave by the patient's bed a lethal drug, which he can take some night if he so desires. But before this, we will have to get over our firmly held idea that for some reason unknown to us, we feel strongly that suicide is a grievous sin.

Dr. Eliot Slater, a renowned British psychiatrist and an active member of The Euthanasia Society, said at the Fifth International Conference for Suicide Prevention in London (1969) that the sick person does indeed have a right to die, be it called "suicide" or "euthanasia." The Euthanasia Society, he said, has produced, with legal help, a notice to help the would-be suicide declare his intentions. One paragraph reads: "I hereby instruct my personal representatives to initiate proceedings against any person who attempts unsuccessfully to resuscitate me, and if the attempt is successful, I shall take action myself."

The idea of legalizing the deliberate termination of an apparently futile existence at the request of the patient has frequently been canvassed, and a survey taken recently among 418 Seattle, Washington physicians to determine their opinions on euthanasia disclosed that those in favor of changing the now-accepted practice of preserving life as long as possible were those who did not often come in contact with dying patients—anesthesiologists, pathologists, psychiatrists, and radiologists (*Journal of the American Medical Association,* January 5, 1970). About one-third of the physicians favored changes in current medical practice which would permit each of the following: (1) negative euthanasia following consent of relatives; (2) positive euthanasia for certain carefully selected patients; or (3) abortion for the convenience of the patient. In the specific instance of patients in a state of chronic uremia, 72 percent of physicians stated that they would exercise negative euthanasia by not performing dialysis on all patients with this disease. Physicians heard requests for negative euthanasia for terminal patients more commonly from family members than from the patients themselves.

At this point a definition of terms is imperative because euthanasia, or "mercy-killing," is a broad term that must be qualified before it can be discussed. Eugenic euthanasia refers to cases of birth monsters, defective children, incurable mental patients and the like. Positive euthanasia is taking actions or instituting procedures which probably will hasten death. Negative euthanasia is omitting procedures and medications from the treatment regimen that probably will extend life.

In 1968, The Euthanasia Society in England, after waging a very aggressive campaign to win support for legalized voluntary euthanasia, prepared "A Draft Bill" for enactment by Parliament. This bill would "authorize physicians to give euthanasia to a patient who is thought on reasonable grounds to be suffering from an irremediable physical condition of a distressing character, and who has, not less than thirty days previously, made a declaration requesting the administration of euthanasia in certain specified circumstances one or more of which has eventuated." The House of Lords on March 25, 1969, rejected this bill. Its sponsor, Lord Raglan, maintained that everyone should be allowed to die when and how they chose and not in a way chosen by someone else. Others denied this and held that all doctors should resist any encouragement or persuasion to kill. And, as in the past, some opposed to the proposal said that doctors were already giving doses of drugs that might shorten life, if they thought the need was indicated. They had gone a long way toward euthanasia and it was doubtful whether it was absolutely necessary to make laws when a good deal of understanding already existed. In fact, Lord Segal, a respected surgeon, told the members of the House of Lords that he had practiced positive and negative euthanasia.

The Euthanasia Society in England has prepared "A Suggested Non-Statutory Declaration" for those who wish to indicate their desire for voluntary euthanasia should the need arise. This states:

The Declaration is made by _____ of _____. *I declare as follows:* If I should at any time suffer from a serious physical illness or impairment thought in my case to be incurable and expected to cause me severe distress or render me incapable to rational existence, then, unless I revoke this declaration or express a wish contrary to its terms, *I request* the administration of whatever quantity of drugs may be required to prevent my feeling pain or distress and, if my suffering cannot be otherwise relieved, to be kept continuously unconscious at a level where dreaming does not take place, *and I decline* to receive any treatment or sustenance designed to prolong my life. *I ask* sympathetically disposed doctors to acknowledge the right of a patient to request certain kinds of treatment and to decline others, and I assure them that if in any situation they think it better for me to die than to survive, I am content to endorse their judgment in advance and in full confidence that they will be acting in my interests to spare me from suffering and ignominy, and also to save my family and friends from anguish I would not want them to endure on my behalf.

Signed

We Testify that the above named declarant signed this declaration in our presence, and appeared to appreciate its significance. We do not know of any pressure being brought upon him/her to make a declaration, and we believe it is made by his/her own wish. So far as we are aware, we do not stand to benefit by the death of the declarant.

Signed by _____ of _____
Signed by _____ of _____

A similar Declaration has been prepared by the Euthanasia Society in the United States and was distributed by this organization in late 1969.

Author's Comment

There is no doubt that there would be less pressure for euthanasia if physicians did not use all the resources at their command to delay death in every patient. Doctors are obligated to prescribe ordinary remedies to sustain life but all doctors do not yet realize that they are not always required to apply extraordinary therapies. In fact, in some instances it could be morally wrong to advise or to employ extraordinary means to prolong life.

Whether a particular treatment is to be classified as ordinary or extraordinary does not depend solely on medical considerations; it also depends on circumstances peculiar to the individual patient. Moralists label as "ordinary" those therapies that are not extraordinary. They define as "extraordinary" whatever here and now is very costly or very unusual or very painful or very difficult or very dangerous, or if the good effects that can be expected from its use are not proportionate to the difficulty and inconvenience that are entailed.

All ill people are obligated to use ordinary means to preserve life, but they are not bound to seek extraordinary treatment except in unusual circumstances. As one moralist puts it: "At times one may be bound in charity to one's dependents or to one's fellow citizens to employ extraordinary means to preserve one's life. In order that such an obligation be present, two conditions must be fulfilled: (1) One is necessary to one's family or fellow-men. (2) The success of the extraordinary means is very probable."

An ill person is not obligated to do what is physically or morally impossible. Hence, he can validly refuse treatment which would entail great suffering, which would overtax the will power and courage of the normal person, or which would financially impoverish his survivors, especially if the anticipated benefits would be of limited value and brief duration. Likewise, a physician, with the patient's consent, may licitly desist from administering treatments that are demonstrably ineffective and be satisfied with alleviating the patient's suffering. No one is required to do what is practically useless. A doctor is not under compulsion to make every effort to prolong every patient's life. Hence, what physicians call negative euthanasia in certain circumstances is not only morally permissible but can be obligatory. In fact, this is not euthanasia and should not be called even negative euthanasia.

Just as the patient has a right to refuse treatment to prolong his life so, too, under certain circumstances he may request a therapy that may endanger or shorten his life even though this is not the cardinal purpose of the treatment. Under the principle of double effect, a person with a widespread, excruciatingly painful disease has a right to ask for whatever drugs, in whatever doses necessary, that will provide relief from his pain and suffering, even though the amount of drug required may be so large as to shorten his life. The doctor prescribes the drug in this manner primarily to alleviate suffering and not to murder by deliberately putting a patient out of his misery. Pope Pius XII stated that analgesic treatment is permissible where the lessening of unbearable pain is achieved by the use of drugs that will shorten life, "provided that no other means exist, and if, in the given circumstances, that action does not prevent the carrying out of other moral and religious duties."

There should be no need for positive euthanasia and there would be no demand for it if doctors acknowledge that it is neither scientific nor humane to use artificial life-sustainers when death is imminent and inevitable and realistic hope of recovery has evaporated. Also there should be no need or demand for positive euthanasia if physicians unhesitatingly administer whatever amount of pain-relieving drugs a dying patient needs. The medical profession has the power to erase any demand for legalized euthanasia. All doctors have to do is apply their skills prudently as they are morally and legally empowered to do. Physicians are not obliged morally or legally to do that which is useless.

No one has the right to be killed and physicians should oppose strenuously any proposal to legalize euthanasia. There are many reasons for this. It would be very dangerous indeed to empower doctors to kill, on demand, the patients they cannot cure. For the conscientious doctor it would be a most difficult and strainful task to decide at what stage of an illness a patient would qualify for euthanasia. It also would be extremely difficult for such a doctor to be sure that the patient knew what he was doing when he requested euthanasia. For the unscrupulous doctor, and there are such, there would have to be very rigorous safeguards against loopholes for murder, and even with these there would be patients at risk for none of us are 100 percent psychologically and morally sound and perversions could creep into the practice of legalized euthanasia. It is better for the community to tie the hands of a good doctor by refusing to legalize voluntary euthanasia, in order to restrain an unscrupulous one from violating the rights of the individual.

Inevitably a physician's judgment is not always right. In his autobiography, *Christiaan Barnard: One Life,* the South African surgeon writes that as a young intern at Groote Schuur hospital, he was a pinprick away from committing euthanasia on a woman who was in extreme agony from terminal cancer. He held a hypodermic needle filled with a solution of morphine over the arm of the dying woman but at the last moment decided, "I was violating not only the laws of social man, but also my own most personal ethic." The following day the patient rallied and went on to live a few more years with the disease in an arrested state.

If voluntary euthanasia were legal, there would be a standing risk of a person consenting to his extinction on an erroneous calculation of his prospects. If it were to become an acknowledged function of the medical profession to end life prematurely, could patients place themselves with complete trust in the care of physicians? A patient's trust in his doctor is important both for his peace of mind and for his recovery.

Many physicians have voiced their opposition to legalizing voluntary euthanasia but few have raised some of the thoughts expressed by Dr. James R. Mathers in a letter to the editor of *The Lancet* (January 3, 1970). Dr. Mathers wrote:

> The notion of voluntary euthanasia implies that a doctor can end a person's life without pain or violence or loss of dignity—and with certainty. How true is this? No doubt some medical procedures are 99 percent effective in 99 percent of cases, but there are few, if any, which carry an absolute guarantee of success in a particular case. How are we to kill people if voluntary euthanasia becomes legal? Will it be by the injection of fifty times the minimum lethal dose of (say) morphine? Or a hundred times? And if, owing to some rare abnormality, or mistake, even this does not kill, what then? In such an event, we may be compelled to use surgical measures: so should these be used only as a last resort, or should the surgeon be called in ab initio? Medical technology has an apparently irreversible tendency towards specialisation. Who would be the specialists in euthanasia? Technique always improves with practice; so does this mean that we have to accept the likelihood that our early attempts at

killing will be unsuccessful, or violent—dysthanasia rather than euthanasia? And will patients consent to euthanasia if they are not assured that it will be administered by the medical attendant they nominate?

Although euthanasia advocates deny it, legalizing voluntary euthanasia could lead to involuntary euthanasia and to a Nazi-style elimination of people judged inferior or undesirable by society. The progress of the law on abortion gives substance to the fear that euthanasia once legalized would be similarly expanded. Anyone attending abortion hearings in the United States or reading the lay and medical press on this subject knows how much the pro-abortion groups have changed their tactics. They are very dissatisfied with the liberal abortion laws and now want abortion on demand or no law governing abortion. They want one individual to be able to decide the fate of another. As Dr. James Fitzgerald has aptly remarked: "The true corollary of abortion on demand is life on demand. Why should not an all-wise government decide who shall live, what number shall be born? Could we not rid our cities and countries of the glut of humanity with a discerning program?" (*Medical Opinion & Review*, January 1970).

Just as abortion advocates have striven to generate an "abortion mentality" through sex education courses for children, euthanasiasts desire to have the idea of "planned death" incorporated into the normal scheme of life. How is this to be brought about? Mary Ross Barrington, a member of the Executive Committee of the Euthanasia Society in England has suggested that school children be asked to write essays on "How I Would Feel If I Had to Die at Midnight," or compositions envisaging why and in what circumstances they propose to end their lives. "An annual visit to a geriatric ward might also be in order," she says. Until we have the "comfort of a death-conditioned society," which may take ten years, Mrs. Barrington says, "I would contend that the true end of education should be to prepare the pupil to learn in the course of life to orientate all knowledge and experience within the framework of a life bounded by decline and death, and to regard a timely and possibly useful death as a summation of the art of living."

Those who have read Walter M. Miller's absorbing science fiction novel *A Canticle for Leibowitz*, know that Mrs. Barrington's idea of educating people to accept "planned death" should the need arise is feasible. In his terrifyingly grim novel Miller recounts the regrowth of the human race after Man nearly erased himself with nuclear weapons. People remembered the billion corpses, the still-born, the monstrous, the dehumanized, and the blind whom survivors begot and sent to asylums. The genetic festering was still with them. Yet, "too much hope for Earth had led men to try to make it Eden." Men learned again how to make nuclear weapons. Knowing what could happen from nuclear explosions, nations tried to prevent their use. But, realizing that a nuclear war could happen, governments passed Radiation Disaster Acts that made mass euthanasia possible. Then it happened. Another nuclear war began. Immediately, fearful of fallout, plans for state-sponsored suicide went into operation. Radio announcers said:

> This station is required by law to broadcast the following announcement twice daily for the duration of the emergency: "The provisions of Public Law 10-WR-3E in no way empower private citizens to administer euthanasia to victims of radiation poisoning. Victims who have been exposed, or who think they have been exposed, to radiation far in excess of the critical dosage must report to the nearest Green Star Relief Station, where a magistrate is empowered to issue a writ of Mori Vult to anyone properly certified as a hopeless case, if the sufferer desires euthanasia. Any victim of radiation who takes his own life in any manner other than that prescribed by law will be considered a suicide, and will jeopardize the right of his heirs and dependents to claim insurance and other radiation relief benefits under the law. Moreover, any citizen who assists such a suicide may be prosecuted for murder. The Radiation Disaster Act authorizes euthanasia only after due process of law. Serious cases of radiation sickness must report to a Green Star Relief. . ."

Euthanasiasts would have science fiction become a reality in the twentieth century with or without the threat of a nuclear war. During the debate on the legalization of voluntary euthanasia in England's House of Lords last year Lord Amulree, who opposed the bill, foresaw, if the law were enacted, a situation wherein certain hospitals might gain a reputation for being "places at which people can get good euthanasia." Miller in his thought-provoking novel described the erection of Mercy Camp Number 18, Green Star, Disaster Cadre Project. This Green Star Camp was picketed by those opposed to euthanasia.

There always will be opposition to man killing man. Human life is sacred and because it is there always will be men who insist that pain is to be eased but that no man has the right to be killed solely to achieve surcease from suffering.

21

Who Lives and Dies?

Frederic Grunberg

ALBANY—Ethical and legal questions faced by health professionals and institutions when parents decide to withhold consent for life-saving treatment of critically ill children are being debated in many quarters.

The guiding principles of some physicians, within the very utilitarian and relativistic morality called situationism, are to support a parental decision to withhold consent for treatment and let an infant die if he happens to be severely mentally retarded or deformed, and if the child is normal to override the parents' decision through judicial intervention.

I do not challenge this utilitarian viewpoint from the absolute belief in the "sanctity of life" but prefer to examine this ethical question from the perspective of justice and fairness, where legal and ethical standards converge.

When a physician supports parents' decisions to deny consent for life-saving surgery and lets an infant, affected, say, by Mongolism die, but seeks judicial intervention to give a blood transfusion to save a "normal" child whose Jehovah Witness parents object to the procedure, what is at issue is whether the two standards of conduct affecting the fate of two humans who cannot participate in a life-or-death decision are just and fair—an issue transcending the emotions and feelings of the other participants in these tragedies, parents and the physician.

Central to the issue of justice is the equal allocation of a right to life to every child whether mentally retarded or of normal intelligence.

Can a just society tolerate two classes of infants and children, one whose right to life is at the mercy of parents' and physicians' decisions, and another whose right is assured through judicial intervention and the full protection of the law?

Obviously no one would suggest that life-saving treatment for all children should depend entirely on the consent of parents. The state cannot withdraw from its obligation as *parens patriae,* or state guardian over the disabled, for all children. On the other hand, if some children are allowed to die through what amounts to negative involuntary euthanasia, they must lack certain qualities that make them less than human.

If the severely retarded children are not human they are not entitled to the equal basic rights assigned to all humans; like animals they may have some protection but their status is not that of a human being.

In our society, mercy killing of animals is not considered unjust because life is not considered a basic right for them; they have other rights such as the right to be protected against cruelty and suffering, but they are not entitled to life as humans are.

The humanness of the severely retarded or deformed is indeed the crux of the matter, and life-or-death decisions by some who consider them less than human is full of perilous consequences. We should not forget that three decades ago hundreds of thousands of defectives and mentally ill were put to death as subhumans because some physicians and philosophers agreed on a new "profile of man."

As a physician who has worked with severely retarded children and adults, I refuse to accept them as less than human. It is true that many of them, especially in state institutions, have been dehumanized through neglect and the failure of their parents and society to meet their needs. But by not allowing them to live, two wrongs will not make a right.

Society in general and physicians in particular do not have any "operable understanding" that the severely retarded and the deformed are not human.

It is thus eminently just and fair that we maintain equally our obligations to save the life of all children, whether defective or not, through ordinary means that offer a reasonable hope of success, even against the wish of their parents, and if necessary through judicial intervention.

22

To Save or Let Die

Richard A. McCormick

On February 24, the son of Mr. and Mrs. Robert H. T. Houle died following court-ordered emergency surgery at Maine Medical Center. The child was born February 9, horribly deformed. His entire left side was malformed; he had no left eye, was practically without a left ear, had a deformed left hand; some of his vertebrae were not fused. Furthermore, he was afflicted with a tracheal esophageal fistula and could not be fed by mouth. Air leaked into his stomach instead of going to the lungs, and fluid from the stomach pushed up into the lungs. As Dr. Andre Hellegers recently noted, "It takes little imagination to think there were further internal deformities" (*Obstetrical and Gynecological News,* April 1974).

As the days passed, the condition of the child deteriorated. Pneumonia set in. His reflexes became impaired and because of poor circulation, severe brain damage was suspected. The tracheal esophageal fistula, the immediate threat to his survival, can be corrected with relative ease by surgery. But in view of the associated complications and deformities, the parents refused their consent to surgery on "Baby Boy Houle." Several doctors in the Maine Medical Center felt differently and took the case to court. Maine Superior Court Judge David G. Roberts ordered the surgery to be performed. He ruled: "At the moment of live birth there does exist a human being entitled to the fullest protection of the law. The most basic right enjoyed by every human being is the right to life itself."

From *JAMA* 229 (July 8, 1974), pp. 172-76. Reprinted by permission of the author and publisher.

"Meaningful Life"

Instances like this happen frequently. In a recent issue of the *New England Journal of Medicine,* Drs. Raymond S. Duff and A. G. M. Campbell reported on 299 deaths in the special-care nursery of the Yale-New Haven Hospital between 1970 and 1972.[1] Of these, 43 (14 percent) were associated with discontinuance of treatment for children with multiple anomalies, trisomy, cardiopulmonary crippling, meningomyelocele, and other central nervous system defects. After careful consideration of each of these 43 infants, parents and physicians in a group decision concluded that the prognosis for "meaningful life" was extremely poor or hopeless, and therefore rejected further treatment. The abstract of the Duff-Campbell report states: "The awesome finality of these decisions, combined with a potential for error in prognosis, made the choice agonizing for families and health professionals. Nevertheless, the issue has to be faced, for not to decide is an arbitrary and potentially devastating decision of default."

In commenting on this study in the *Washington Post* (October 28, 1973), Dr. Lawrence K. Pickett, chief-of-staff at the Yale-New Haven Hospital, admitted that allowing hopelessly ill patients to die "is accepted medical practice." He continued: "This is nothing new. It's just being talked about now."

It has been talked about, it is safe to say, at least since the publicity associated with the famous "Johns Hopkins Case" some three years ago.[2] In this instance, an infant was born with Down syndrome and duodenal atresia. The blockage is reparable by relatively easy surgery. However, after consultation with spiritual advisors, the parents refused permission for this corrective surgery, and the child died by starvation in the hospital after fifteen days. For to feed him by mouth in this condition would have killed him. Nearly everyone who has commented on this case has disagreed with the decision.

It must be obvious that these instances—and they are frequent—raise the most agonizing and delicate moral problems. The problem is best seen in the ambiguity of the term "hopelessly ill." This used to and still may refer to lives that cannot be saved, that are irretrievably in the dying process. It may also refer to lives that can be saved and sustained, but in a wretched, painful, or deformed condition. With regard to infants, the problem is, which infants, if any, should be allowed to die? On what grounds or according to what criteria, as determined by whom? Or again, is there a point at which a life that can be saved is not "meaningful life," as the medical community so often phrases the question? If our past experience is any hint of the future, it is safe to say that public discussion of such controversial issues will quickly collapse into slogans such as "There is no such thing as a life not worth saving" or "Who is the physician to play God?" We saw and continue to see this far too frequently in the abortion debate. We are experiencing it in the euthanasia discussion. For instance, "death with dignity" translates for many into a death that is fast, clean, painless. The trouble with slogans is that they do not aid in the discovery of truth; they co-opt this discovery and promulgate it rhetorically, often only thinly disguising a good number of questionable value judgments in the process. Slogans are not tools for analysis and enlightenment; they are weapons for ideological battle.

Thus far, the ethical discussion of these truly terrifying decisions has been less than fully satisfactory. Perhaps this is to be expected since the problems have only recently come to public attention. In a companion article to the Duff-Campbell report, Dr. Anthony Shaw of the Pediatric Division of the Department of Surgery, University of Virginia Medical Center, Charlottesville, speaks of solutions "based on the circumstances of each case rather than by means of a dogmatic formula approach."[3] Are these really the only options available to us? Shaw's statement makes it appear that the ethical alternatives are narrowed to dogmatism (which imposes a formula that prescinds from circumstances) and pure concretism (which denies the possibility or usefulness of any guidelines).

Are Guidelines Possible?

Such either-or extremism is understandable. It is easy for the medical profession, in its fully justified concern with the terrible concreteness of these problems and with the issue of who makes these decisions, to trend away from any substantive guidelines. As *Time* remarked in reporting these instances: "Few, if any, doctors are willing to establish guidelines for determining which babies should receive lifesaving surgery or treatment and which should not" (*Time,* March 25, 1974). On the other hand, moral theologians, in their fully justified concern to avoid total normlessness and arbitrariness wherein the right is "discovered," or really "created," only in and by brute decision, can easily be insensitive to the moral relevance of the raw experience, of the conflicting tensions and concerns provoked through direct cradle-side contact with human events and persons.

But is there no middle course between sheer concretism and dogmatism? I believe there is. Dr. Franz J. Ingelfinger, editor of the *New England Journal of Medicine,* in an editorial on the Duff-Campbell—Shaw articles, concluded, even if somewhat reluctantly: "Society, ethics, institutional attitudes and committees can provide the broad guidelines, but the onus of decision-making ultimately falls on the doctor in whose care the child has been put."[4] Similarly, Frederick Carney of Southern Methodist University, Dallas, and the Kennedy Center for Bioethics stated of these cases: "What is obviously needed is the development of substantive standards to inform parents and physicians who must make such decisions" (*Washington Post,* March 20, 1974).

"Broad guidelines," "substantive standards." There is the middle course, and it is the task of a community broader than the medical community. A guideline is not a slide rule that makes the decision. It is far less than that. But it is far more than the concrete decision of the parents and physician, however seriously and conscientiously this is made. It is more like a light in a room, a light that allows the individual objects to be seen in the fullness of their context. Concretely, if there are certain infants that we agree ought to be saved in spite of illness or deformity, and if there are certain infants that we agree should be allowed to die, then there is a line to be drawn. And if there is a line to be drawn, there ought to be some criteria, even if very general, for doing this. Thus, if nearly every commentator has disagreed with the Hopkins decision, should we not be able to distill from such consensus some general wisdom that will inform and guide future decisions? I think so.

This task is not easy. Indeed, it is so harrowing that the really tempting thing is to run from it. The most sensitive, balanced, and penetrating study of the Hopkins case that I have seen is that of the University of Chicago's James Gustafson. Gustafson disagreed with the decision of the Hopkins physicians to deny surgery to the mongoloid infant. In summarizing his dissent, he notes: "Why would I draw the line on a different side of mongolism than the physicians did? While reasons can be given, one must recognize that there are intuitive elements, grounded in beliefs and profound feelings, that enter into particular judgments of this sort." He goes on to criticize the assessment made of the child's intelligence as too simplistic, and he proposes a much broader perspective on the meaning of suffering than seemed to have operated in the Hopkins decision. I am in full agreement with Gustafson's reflections and conclusions. But ultimately, he does not tell us where he would draw the line or why, only where he would *not,* and why.

This is very helpful already, and perhaps it is all that can be done. Dare we take the next step, the combination and analysis of such negative judgments to extract from them the positive criterion or criteria inescapably operative in them? Or more startlingly, dare we *not* if these decisions are already being made? Gustafson is certainly right in saying that we cannot always establish perfectly rational accounts and norms for our decisions. But I believe we must never cease trying, in fear and trembling to be sure. Otherwise, we have exempted these decisions in principle from the one critique and control that protects against abuse. Exemption of this sort is the root of all exploitation whether personal or political. Briefly, if we must face the frightening task of making quality-of-life judgments—and we must—then we must face the difficult task of building criteria for these judgments.

Facing Responsibility

What has brought us to this position of awesome responsibility? Very simply, the sophistication of modern medicine. Contemporary resuscitation and life-sustaining devices have brought a remarkable change in the state of the question. Our duties toward the care and preservation of life have been traditionally stated in terms of the use of ordinary and extraordinary means. For the moment and for purposes of brevity, we may say that, morally speaking, ordinary means are those whose use does not entail grave hardships to the patient. Those that would involve such hardship are extraordinary. Granted the relativity of these terms and the frequent difficulty of their application, still the distinction has had an honored place in medical ethics and medical practice. Indeed, the distinction was recently reiterated by the House of Delegates of the American Medical Association in a policy statement. After disowning intentional killing (mercy killing), the AMA statement continues: "The cessation of the employment of extraordinary means to prolong the life of the body when there is irrefutable evidence that biological death is imminent is the decision of the patient and/or his immediate family. The advice and judgment of the physician should be freely available to the patient and/or his immediate family" (*JAMA* 227:728, 1974).

This distinction can take us just so far—and thus the change in the state of the question. The contemporary problem is precisely that the question no longer concerns only those for whom "biological death is imminent" in the sense of the AMA statement. Many infants who would have died a decade ago, whose "biological death was imminent," can be saved. Yesterday's failures are today's successes. Contemporary medicine with its team approaches, staged surgical techniques, monitoring capabilities, ventilatory support systems, and other methods, can keep almost anyone alive. This has tended gradually to shift the problem from the means to reverse the dying process to the quality of the life sustained and preserved. The questions, "Is this means too hazardous or difficult to use" and "Does this measure only prolong the patient's dying," while still useful and valid, now often become "Granted that we can easily save the life, what kind of life are we saving?" This is a quality of life judgment. And we fear it. And certainly we should. But with increased power goes increased responsibility. Since we have the power, we must face the responsibility.

A Relative Good

In the past, the Judeo-Christian tradition has attempted to walk a balanced middle path between medical vitalism (that preserves life at any cost) and medical pessimism (that kills when life seems frustrating, burdensome, "useless"). Both of these extremes root in an identical idolatry of life—an attitude that, at least by inference, views death as an unmitigated, absolute evil, and life as the absolute good. The middle course that has structured Judeo-Christian attitudes is that life is indeed a basic and precious good, but a good to be preserved precisely as the condition of other values. It is these other values and possibilities that found the duty to preserve physical life and also dictate the limits of this duty. In other words, life is a relative good, and the duty to preserve it a limited one. These limits have always been stated in terms of the *means* required to sustain life. But if the implications of this middle position are unpacked a bit, they will allow us, perhaps, to adapt to the type of quality-of-life judgment we are now called on to make without tumbling into vitalism or a utilitarian pessimism.

A beginning can be made with a statement of Pope Pius XII in an allocution to physicians delivered November 24, 1957.[5] After noting that we are normally obliged to use only ordinary means to preserve life, the Pontiff stated: "A more strict obligation would be too burdensome for most men and would render the attainment of the higher, more important good too difficult. Life, death, all temporal activities are in fact subordinated to spiritual ends." Here it would be helpful to ask two questions. First, what are these spiritual ends, this "higher, more important good?" Second, how is its attainment rendered too difficult by insisting on the use of extraordinary means to preserve life?

The first question must be answered in terms of love of God and neighbor. This sums up briefly the meaning, substance, and consummation of life from a Judeo-Christian perspective. What is or can easily be missed is that these two loves are not separable. St. John wrote: "If any man says I love God and hates his brother, he is a liar. For he who loves not his brother, whom he sees, how can he love God whom he does not see?" (1 John 4:20-21). This means that our love of neighbor is in some very real sense our love of God. The good our love wants to do Him and to which He enables us, can be done only for the neighbor, as Karl Rahner has so forcefully argued. It is in others that God demands to be recognized and loved. If this is true, it means that, in Judeo-Christian perspective, the meaning, substance, and consummation of life is found in human *relationships,* and the qualities of justice, respect, concern, compassion, and support, that surround them.

Second, how is the attainment of this "higher, more important (than life) good" rendered "too difficult" by life-supports that are gravely burdensome? One who must support his life with disproportionate effort focuses the time, attention, energy, and resources of himself and others not precisely on relationships, but on maintaining the condition of relationships. Such concentration easily becomes overconcentration and distorts one's view of and weakens one's pursuit of the very relational goods that define our growth and flourishing. The importance of relationships gets lost in the struggle for survival. The very Judeo-Christian meaning of life is seriously jeopardized when undue and unending effort must go into its maintenance.

I believe an analysis similar to this is implied in traditional treatises on preserving life. The illustrations of grave hardship (rendering the means to preserve life extraordinary and nonobligatory) are instructive, even if they are outdated in some of their particulars. Older moralists often referred to the hardship of moving to another climate or country. As the late Gerald Kelly, S.J. noted of this instance:

> They [the classical moral theologians] spoke of other inconveniences, too: e.g., of moving to another climate or another country to preserve one's life. For people whose lives were, so to speak, rooted in the land, and whose native town or village was as dear as life itself, and for whom, moreover, travel was always difficult and often dangerous—for such people, moving to another country or climate was a truly great hardship, and more than God would demand as a "reasonable" means of preserving one's health and life.[6]

Similarly, if the financial cost of life-preserving care was crushing, that is, if it would create grave hardships for oneself or one's family, it was considered extraordinary and nonobligatory. Or again, the grave inconvenience of living with a badly mutilated body was viewed, along with other factors (such as pain in preanesthetic days, uncertainty of success), as constituting the means extraordinary. Even now, the contemporary moralist, M. Zalba, S.J., states that no one is obliged to preserve his life when the cost is "a most oppressive convalescence" (*molestissima convalescentia*).[7]

The Quality of Life

In all of these instances—instances where the life could be saved—the discussion is couched in terms of the means necessary to preserve life. But often enough it is the kind of, the quality of the life thus saved (painful, poverty-stricken and deprived, away from home and friends, oppressive) that establishes the means as extraordinary. *That* type of life would be an excessive hardship for the individual. It would distort and jeopardize his grasp on the overall meaning of life. Why? Because, it can be argued, human relationships—which are the very possibility of growth in love of God and neighbor—would be so threatened, strained, or submerged that they would no longer function as the heart and meaning of the individual's life as they should. Something other than the "higher, more important good" would occupy first place.

Life, the condition of other values and achievements, would usurp the place of these and become itself the ultimate value. When that happens, the value of human life has been distorted out of context.

In his *Morals in Medicine,* Thomas O'Donnell, S.J., hinted at an analysis similar to this. Noting that life is a relative, not an absolute good, he asks: Relative to what? His answer moves in two steps. First, he argues that life is the fundamental natural good God has given to man, "the fundamental context in which all other goods which God has given man as means to the end proposed to him, must be exercised." Second, since this is so, the relativity of the good of life consists in the effort required to preserve this fundamental context and "the potentialities of the other goods that still remain to be worked out within that context."[8]

Can these reflections be brought to bear on the grossly malformed infant? I believe so. Obviously there is a difference between having a terribly mutilated body as the result of surgery, and having a terribly mutilated body from birth. There is also a difference between a long, painful, oppressive convalescence resulting from surgery, and a life that is from birth one long, painful, oppressive convalescence. Similarly, there is a difference between being plunged into poverty by medical expenses and being poor without ever incurring such expenses. However, is there not also a similarity? Cannot these conditions, whether caused by medical intervention or not, equally absorb attention and energies to the point where the "higher, more important good" is simply too difficult to attain? It would appear so. Indeed, is this not precisely why abject poverty (and the systems that support it) is such an enormous moral challenge to us? It simply dehumanizes.

Life's potentiality for other values is dependent on two factors, those external to the individual, and the very condition of the individual. The former we can and must change to maximize individual potential. That is what social justice is all about. The latter we sometimes cannot alter. It is neither inhuman nor unchristian to say that there comes a point where an individual's condition itself represents the negation of any truly human—i.e., relational—potential. When that point is reached, is not the best treatment no treatment? I believe that the *implications* of the traditional distinction between ordinary and extraordinary means point in this direction.

In this tradition, life is not a value to be preserved in and for itself. To maintain that would commit us to a form of medical vitalism that makes no human or Judeo-Christian sense. It is a value to be preserved precisely as a condition for other values, and therefore insofar as these other values remain attainable. Since these other values cluster around and are rooted in human relationships, it seems to follow that life is a value to be preserved only insofar as it contains some potentiality for human relationships. When in human judgment this potentiality is totally absent or would be, because of the condition of the individual, totally subordinated to the mere effort for survival, that life can be said to have achieved its potential.

Human Relationships

If these reflections are valid, they point in the direction of a guideline that may help in decisions about sustaining the lives of grossly deformed and deprived infants. That guideline is the potential for human relationships associated with the infant's condition. If that potential is simply nonexistent or would be utterly submerged and undeveloped in the mere struggle to survive, that life has achieved its potential. There are those who will want to continue to say that some terribly deformed infants may be allowed to die *because* no extraordinary means need be used. Fair enough. But they should realize that the term "extraordinary" has been so relativized to the condition of the patient that it is this condition that is decisive. The means is extraordinary because the infant's condition is extraordinary. And if that is so, we must face this fact head-on—and discover the substantive standard that allows us to say this of some infants, but not of others.

Here several caveats are in order. First, this guideline is not a detailed rule that preempts decisions; for relational capacity is not subject to mathematical analysis but to human judgment. However, it is the task of physicians to provide some more concrete categories or presumptive biological symptoms for this human judgment. For instance, nearly all would very likely agree that the anencephalic infant is without relational potential. On the other hand, the same cannot be said of the mongoloid infant. The task ahead is to attach relational potential to presumptive biological symptoms for the gray area between such extremes. In other words, individual decisions will remain the anguishing onus of parents in consultation with physicians.

Second, because this guideline is precisely that, mistakes will be made. Some infants will be judged in all sincerity to be devoid of any meaningful relational potential when that is actually not quite the case. This risk of error should not lead to abandonment of decisions; for that is to walk away from the human scene. Risk of error means only that we must proceed with great humility, caution, and tentativeness. Concretely, it means that if err we must at times, it is better to err on the side of life—and therefore to tilt in that direction.

Third, it must be emphasized that allowing some infants to die does not imply that "some lives are valuable, others not" or that "there is such a thing as a life not worth living." Every human being, regardless of age or condition, is of incalculable worth. The point is not, therefore, whether this or that individual has value. Of course he has, or rather *is* a value. The only point is whether this undoubted value has any potential at all, in continuing physical survival, for attaining a share, even if reduced, in the "higher, more important good." This is not a question about the inherent value of the individual. It is a question about whether this worldly existence will offer such a valued individual any hope of sharing those values for which physical life is the fundamental condition. Is not the only alternative an attitude that supports mere physical life as long as possible with every means?

Fourth, this whole matter is further complicated by the fact that this decision is being made for someone else. Should not the decision on whether life is to be supported or not be left to the individual? Obviously, wherever possible. But there is nothing inherently objectionable in the fact that parents with physicians must make this decision at some point for infants. Parents must make many crucial decisions for children. The only concern is that the decision not be shaped out of the utilitarian perspectives so deeply sunk into the consciousness of the contemporary world. In a highly technological culture, an individual is always in danger of being valued for his function, what he can do, rather than for who he is.

It remains, then, only to emphasize that these decisions must be made in terms of the child's good, this alone. But that good, as fundamentally a relational good, has many dimensions. Pius XII, in speaking of the duty to preserve life, noted that this duty "derives from well-ordered charity, from submission to the

Creator, from social justice, as well as from devotion towards his family." All of these considerations pertain to that "higher, more important good." If that is the case with the duty to preserve life, then the decision not to preserve life must likewise take all of these into account in determining what is for the child's good.

Any discussion of this problem would be incomplete if it did not repeatedly stress that it is the pride of Judeo-Christian tradition that the weak and defenseless, the powerless and unwanted, those whose grasp on the goods of life is most fragile—that is, those whose potential is real but reduced—are cherished and protected as our neighbor in greatest need. Any application of a general guideline that forgets this is but a racism of the adult world profoundly at odds with the gospel, and eventually corrosive of the humanity of those who ought to be caring and supporting as long as that care and support has human meaning. It has meaning as long as there is hope that the infant will, in relative comfort, be able to experience our caring and love. For when this happens, both we and the child are sharing in that "greater, more important good."

Were not those who disagreed with the Hopkins decision saying, in effect, that for the infant, involved human relationships were still within reach and would not be totally submerged by survival? If that is the case, it is potential for relationships that is at the heart of these agonizing decisions.

Notes

1. Raymond S. Duff and A.G.M. Campbell, "Moral and Ethical Dilemmas in the Special-care Nursery," *New England Journal of Medicine* 289 (1973), pp. 890-94.

2. James M. Gustafson, "Mongolism, Parental Desires, and the Right to Life," *Perspectives on Biological Medicine* 16 (1973), pp. 529-59.

3. Anthony Shaw, "Dilemmas of 'Informed' Consent in Children," *New England Journal of Medicine* 289 (1973), p. 885-90.

4. Franz J. Ingelfinger, "Bedside Ethics for the Hopeless Case," *New England Journal of Medicine* 289 (1973), p. 914.

5. Pope Pius XII, *Acta Apostolicae Sedis* 49 (1957), p. 1031-32.

6. Gerald Kelly, *Medico-Moral Problems* (St. Louis: Catholic Hospital Association of the United States and Canada, 1957), p. 132.

7. M. Zalba, *Theologiae Moralis Summa* (Madrid: La Editorial Catolica, 1957), vol. 2, p. 71.

8. Thomas O'Donnell, *Morals in Medicine* (Westminster, Md.: Newman Press, 1957), p. 66.

23

The Living Will—
and the Will to Live

David Dempsey

A few years ago, at a conference on death and dying at Columbia
Presbyterian Medical Center, I sat next to an attractive young
woman whose name tag read, "Hi! I'm Betty L—." During the
coffee break, as we talked, she showed me a "Living Will"
requesting that doctors take responsibility for doing what she
herself would be unable to do if she became hopelessly ill—terminate her life. Although the will was not binding, she hoped that
when "her time came" they would take it seriously.

Addressed to "My family, my physician, my clergyman, my
lawyer," this legal-looking document expressed the wish that "if
there is no reasonable expectation of my recovery from physical
or mental disability, I, Betty L—, be allowed to die and not be
kept alive by artifical means or heroic measures. . . . I ask that drugs
be mercifully administered to me for terminal suffering even if
they hasten the moment of death."

It was hard to visualize that vivacious woman hooked up to the
awesome machinery of intensive care—the catheters, respirators,
monitors, bottles and intravenous tubes by which a dying person
can be kept alive. But her fear of this possibility, I found out, is
not unusual. At least 300,000 model wills have been distributed
by churches, doctors and even schools, and no one knows how
many people have written their own. When Abigail Van Buren
described the will in her widely syndicated "Dear Abby" column,
the Euthanasia Educational Council—prime supplier of the document—received 50,000 requests representing every state in the
union.

"Right to Die" educational kits are supplied by the Euthanasia
Council to schools throughout the country, down to grade seven;

TO MY FAMILY, MY PHYSICIAN, MY LAWYER, MY CLERGYMAN
TO ANY MEDICAL FACILITY IN WHOSE CARE I HAPPEN TO BE
TO ANY INDIVIDUAL WHO MAY BECOME RESPONSIBLE FOR MY HEALTH, WELFARE OR
AFFAIRS

Death is as much a reality as birth, growth, maturity and old age—it is the one certainty of life. If the time comes when I, _____ can no longer take part in decisions for my own future, let this statement stand as an expression of my wishes, while I am still of sound mind.

If the situation should arise in which there is no reasonable expectation of my recovery from physical or mental disability, I request that I be allowed to die and not be kept alive by artificial means or "heroic measures". I do not fear death itself as much as the indignities of deterioration, dependence and hopeless pain. I, therefore, ask that medication be mercifully administered to me to alleviate suffering even though this may hasten the moment of death.

This request is made after careful consideration. I hope you who care for me will feel morally bound to follow its mandate. I recognize that this appears to place a heavy responsibility upon you, but it is with the intention of relieving you of such responsibility and of placing it upon myself in accordance with my strong convictions, that this statement is made.

Signed _____

Date _____

Witness _____

Witness _____

Copies of this request have been given to _____

_____

_____

_____

and for $55, a 56-minute "Right to Die" film, in color, can be rented by organizations. Bills to legalize voluntary euthanasia have been introduced in a number of state legislatures (none, however, have been approved); and although doctors in general are wary of committing themselves in public, many admittedly "pull the plug"—or have the nurse trip over it—when there is no hope of recovery. Dr. Walter W. Sackett, Jr., a Miami, Florida, general practitioner—if not the Semmelweiss of geriatric medicine, at least its Billy Mitchell—boasts that he has allowed "hundreds of patients" to die by withholding treatment, and sees no other satisfactory answer to the problem of prolonged terminal illness.

The right to die hardly competes with Women's Lib for public attention, nor is it as controversial as abortion; to many people, however, it represents one of the last unresolved issues in the battle for human rights. Many civil libertarians, for example, contending that everyone is entitled to control over his own body, assert that one's mode of dying should be as privileged a part of one's life-style as long hair, clothes and sex. Under the Constitution, they argue, the right to die is as inalienable as the right to live.

The slogan of the movement, "Death with Dignity," implies a rejection of the paraphernalia by which a terminal patient is kept alive, usually at great cost to his family and in isolation from them. Such "intensive care"—so the argument goes—is often less for the patient's benefit than the physician's; it reduces the person to an object, prolongs dying (rather than living) and, for many people, needlessly makes death a psychologically, if not physically, anguishing experience.

This upsurge of interest in death with dignity, however, has obscured an undercurrent of doubt, and even outright opposition, on the part of clergymen, doctors and legal experts who question whether dying is quite that simple, or that it is a "right" that can be isolated from society's right to protect human life. Some of the movement's earliest ideologists are also beginning to have second thoughts about specific directions the movement is taking.

"The Living Will is hard for me to swallow," says Dr. Austin H. Kutscher, a professor of dentistry at Columbia Presbyterian Medical School and president of the Foundation of Thanatology, a New York-based educational and research organization that promotes a broader understanding of the "new" dying among both professionals and laymen. "An individual signs it under circumstances when he is not concerned with his own death. It becomes operative at a time when he is 100 percent involved. There's no provision for canceling out." (Mindful of this criticism, the Euthanasia Council has since amended its will by suggesting that signers redate it once a year if their wishes are unchanged).

For Dr. Robert Kastenbaum, a research psychologist and gerontologist who has written widely on the subject of dying, promoting the right to die is a "cop-out" that gives the medical profession an excuse to limit, rather than improve, care of the dying. "It's much easier to talk about mercy killing," he says, "than to try to add comfort and value to a terminal life."

Critics of the right to die admit there are times when human life is so meaningless that death may be preferable. A man or woman with irreversible brain damage who remains hostage to a heart-lung machine can hardly be said to "live" at all. Similarly, the moribund old person is psychologically if not physically, dead, although it is unlikely that he suffers. For these patients, "pulling the plug" may be the only solution. A matter of medical judgment, often performed with the family's consent, it is a perfectly legal as well as merciful way of letting "natural" death take over from the machines. It does not, however, expedite what otherwise would not have occurred.

Such clear-cut instances, however, represent a small number of problem deaths and, in any case, medicine already handles them with discretion and mercy. The real danger, these opponents point out, lies in an overly simplistic attitude toward dying in general, primarily the view that a "good" death is something that can be anticipated and managed. What may appear to be an individual right, moreover, is actually entwined in a number of social relationships. Before a verdict can be rendered, they say, at least four crucial aspects of the problem need to be examined:

1. Does a person, in fact, have a constitutional right to die? If so, is the right always in his best interests?

2. Does death by choice represent medicine's best answer to the admittedly difficult question of incurable and/or terminal illness?

3. Does society have an investment in human life—and the concept of its sacredness—that overrides the individual, if not legally, at least morally? (Conversely, does the notion of "easy death" give society a dangerous weapon to regulate population in a world burdened with too many unproductive people?)

4. Does the right to die, in effect, sanction unconscious, self-destructive impulses in people? Is it another escapist symptom in a world looking for easy answers to the human dilemma?

The U.S. Supreme Court has never ruled on a case involving the right to die; its constitutional standing, therefore, is not certain. Lower courts have almost always ruled in favor of the individual when it can be shown that he or she is a mentally competent adult.

A few years ago, in Miami, Florida, Judge David Popper, of the Dade County Circuit Court, declared that a Cuban refugee, Mrs. Carmen Martinez, had the legal right to refuse continued treatment for hemolytic anemia. The treatment was extremely painful—"cutdowns," or surgical incisions, were made into the skin so that blood could be forced into her veins. After two months of this, Mrs. Martinez begged her doctors to let her die. Uncertain of their own rights, they went to court and received approval to stop treatment. "This woman has a right not to be hurt," Judge Popper ruled. "She has a right to live or die in dignity." The transfusions were stopped and one day later Mrs. Martinez died.

To avoid the need for adjudicating every questionable case that might arise, some 1,700 New York State physicians petitioned the Legislature several years ago to permit voluntary euthanasia, with safeguards. To exercise this right to die, however, the patient was required to make solemn application on a prescribed form in the presence of two witnesses. The sponsorship of two doctors was also necessary. An independent referee would then interview the person, to be followed by a five-day waiting period in which he could change his mind. Final decision was to be made by a court, which had three days to act. If the petition was denied, the patient had the right of appeal.

Clearly, this was no road to a quiet and easy death. For all practical purposes, the dying person was required to fight a lawsuit, in the face of which, one lawyer commented, "it might really be easier for him to hang on and make the best of it." Nevertheless, a streamlined, somewhat less cumbersome version of this bill has been redrafted and is awaiting introduction in the next session of the Legislature.

Critics of such legislation point out that the real problem is not the mentally competent adult who suffers an incurable and painful disease, but the unconscious or confused patient who is in no condition to make his wishes known and who, in fact, may not be suffering at all. A California doctor cites a patient with irreversible brain damage who was kept "alive" for eight years with a catheter in his bladder. "Every eight hours a nurse would poke a tube down his throat and shoot some food in. . ." Three special nurses were required and the cost of "treatment" for the period amounted to almost $200,000.

Dr. Richard Restak, writing in the *Washington Post,* describes the case of a young Pennsylvania man, Robert Carter, who was injured in an automobile accident in 1966 and has been unconscious ever since. At one point, six years after the accident, Carter's father decided that it was time to quit and, with the doctor's consent, plans were made to stop the intravenous feeding. Then, overnight, the father changed his mind. He was willing to go on with his twenty-seven-year-old son in an unconscious state.

The mother of a man I know is senile, although otherwise sound at eighty-nine. Recently, she fell and broke her hip. Surgery, if she survived it, would prolong her life for months, if not years. The family, not the mother, must make the decision. "How can I ask her if she wants to go on living," her son says, "when she doesn't know who I am?"

Advocates of death by consent say these problems would be taken care of by the Living Will; this is doubtful, however, since the will at present has no legal force. Professor Cyril Means of the New York University Law School, an expert on constitutional law, suggests solving the question by a Committee of the Person to do for the unconscious or incompetent patient what the law already provides for in the management of his personal affairs—in a word, death (or life) by committee. Some hospitals already employ group decisions to this end. Family, clergy, medical staff and possibly a psychiatrist are brought in to render a verdict when the patient cannot speak for himself.

But, in the opinion of many doctors, the risks inherent in choosing death may be even greater when the patient *can* speak for himself. The option of refusing treatment can seldom be separated from the subjective context of the illness. In short, the patient may not necessarily know his true condition. He may think he is dying when, in fact, he has good chances for recovery. He may be in a postoperative depression. He may worry about the financial burden he is imposing on his family. None of these reasons justify the termination of treatment. Doctors tend to resist such pleas, even though the courts now seem to side with the patient. Unfortunately, a strictly construed "right to die" includes the right to be mistaken. Worse, it is a mistake that, once made, cannot be corrected.

Although he is a member of the Euthanasia Council's Medical Advisory Committee, Dr. Avery Weisman, a Boston psychiatrist and professor at Harvard Medical School, has never signed a Living Will. "I don't want someone pulling the plug on me because they need the bed," he says, adding, "I know some doctors that I wouldn't want in charge of telling me the time of day, let along the time to die."

For most physicians, however, it is not the truly terminal case that creates a dilemma. Far more common are patients who suffer from such prolonged illnesses as cancer, coronary disease and kidney failure, as well as the elderly man or woman who "lingers on" with a multiplicity of ailments long after death has started rapping at the door. For the former group, modern drugs not only control pain but can make possible an extended life span that is useful and meaningful to the person. They also hold out the promise of a cure. Pernicious anemia and diabetes mellitus were once "incurable" diseases. Blood infections were often fatal, as was pneumonia. Effective treatment of such diseases, once considered "extraordinary," is now commonplace.

The "right to die," physicians point out, comes at a time when breakthroughs in medical progress have never been brighter, and when society is placing a renewed value on the lives of the elderly. In any case, they add, it is not machine medicine that allows more people to live to be old and feeble, but antibiotics, a healthier environment, improved nutrition and better medical care in general—and no one proposes to eliminate these.

Nor is intensive care always the chamber of horrors that death-with-dignity euthusiasts accuse it of being. It is the outsider's unfamiliarity with this equipment, medical specialists contend, that makes it resemble a torture rack. The patient who has difficulty breathing, or who cannot swallow, would be more uncomfortable without it even in a terminal situation. "Dignity," writes Dr. Franklin H. Epstein of the Harvard Medical School, "lies in the patient's fight for life and in his struggle to maintain human contact, in the feeling that someone cares about him and is trying to help him." Withdrawing treatment doesn't necessarily mean that a patient will die with dignity; it means that he will probably die quicker.

There is some evidence, in fact, that intensive care, in spite of its frightening apparatus, reassures the seriously ill person and strengthens his will to live. Dr. Thomas Hackett and a group of colleagues studied a number of coronary patients in the intensive care unit at Massachusetts General Hospital in Boston. They found that those who accepted the "machines" most readily, and by implication denied that they might die, were most likely to recover. Patients with the least denial—8 percent of the sample— accounted for 50 percent of the mortality in the unit. To conclude that an illness might be fatal, hence subject to withdrawal of treatment, can weaken the will to live. At one hospital in London devoted to the treatment of the terminally ill, an average of 10 percent of all patients so diagnosed are regularly discharged—to live months, and even years, longer.

But if a person is in pain, and hopelessly ill, how much suffering must he face before he is allowed to die, and who is to be the judge? If the family, which members? What if they disagree? What hidden death-wishes might be buried in their decision? If no family is available, what are the risks of death by committee? Age itself might be the determinant. When a number of physicians in Great Britain were asked to propose a point beyond which a dying person should not be resuscitated, suggestions varied from sixty-five to eighty years! The lower age was frequently cited because that is presumably the last year of productivity.

But an attitude which encourages those over sixty-five to bow out gracefully and a little sooner than they might ordinarily choose, becomes one more booby trap in the minefield of old age. Unproductive, often burdensome to others, they are presented with a "right" which may look more like a duty. Social critics of the Living Will think that it may operate as a subtle document of self-rejection. Dorothea Jaeger and Leo W. Simmons, in their book, *The Aged Ill,* state that, because the elderly "see an image of themselves as not useful citizens, [they] are likely to go tacitly along with euthanasia programs."

But if the 25,000 members of the Euthanasia Council are typical, by far the largest bloc of support for voluntary death comes from the middleaged. These people are apparently signing up for what they consider to be a "good death" for themselves when they get old. The indications are, however, that at least some of the most enthusiastic supporters of the Living Will change their minds when the moment of truth arrives.

Mrs. Arthur E. Morgan, wife of the former head of the TVA, once wrote, in a letter that has been widely circulated by church groups and others, that "one should be allowed to drink the hemlock in some dignified and simple way." Although she later became blind, largely deaf and senile, she herself did not reach for the hemlock, nor was it passed to her. A family conference called to discuss the matter decided against it, and Mrs. Morgan died in a nursing home at ninety-four.

Indeed, there is considerable evidence that people are less likely to want to die when they are old than when they were young and "useful." In 1972, the Gannett newspaper chain assigned a reporter, John Dalmas, to interview residents of Rockland County, N.Y., on the subject of euthanasia. He found the most ardent supporters of death by consent to be those who had the least contact with elderly and the ill. At a Jewish home for convalescents, residents, who ranged in age from sixty-three to eighty-five, generally opposed voluntary death. "Talk to some young people," a man in his sixties told Mr. Dalmas. "They'll be glad to talk about it. You're not going to get much interest here." Mr. Dalmas did talk to young people and found that the most enthusiastic supporters of the right to die were teen-agers.

Thomas Bane, a chaplain at Grasslands Hospital in Westchester County, says that in his three years there, and in ten years as a parish priest, no one has ever begged him to hasten death. "A woman in my parish had a stroke," he reported, "and as far as people could tell she was completely comatose. They would talk in front of her as if she weren't there. I'd visit and hold her hand. Before she died, she partially recovered and told me she knew we were there. She appreciated what I had done. There was some kind of life experience that had meaning for her."

More than twenty million persons in the United States are sixty-five or over—between 10 and 11 percent of the population; with a lowering of the birthrate in the next few decades, this proportion is expected to rise to 15 percent. Because many of these people will be economically if not socially superfluous, death for the old may be viewed in terms of Malthusian pressures as well as merciful release. Although not pleading for euthanasia, Dr. Charles K. Hofling, a psychiatrist, thinks it "unlikely that the termination of individual human life. . . can be left indefinitely to 'natural causes.' People will have to decide when to let natural causes take over."

With Medicare and Medicaid paying for a large part of terminal care, financial reasons alone may force a cut-off point for the impecunious patient that does not reflect his true medical condition. It is probably no coincidence that the Euthanasia Council's most numerous supporters are found in California, or that the most persistent efforts to legalize euthanasia take place in Florida. Both states have a disproportionate number of old people among their populations.

"In my opinion," Dr. Alvin I. Goldfarb of Mount Sinai Hospital told a Right to Die symposium sponsored by the Group for the Advancement of Psychiatry, "the [current] preoccupation with death is a sign of ultraconservatism and authoritarianism. . ." One danger of this preoccupation, he added, is that "controlling forces within the establishment may decide for the living that their lives are considered of little value, that they may be killed or allowed to die at government whim." In Germany, in the 1930s, thousands of mental incompetents and "useless eaters" were put to death by psychiatrists acting quite independent of Hitler. No one in this country seriously proposes such an approach, yet voluntary death might be even more insidious—democracy's use of a civil liberty to encourage what it cannot do by fiat.

Psychiatrists who work with dying patients point out that a person brings to his death all the conflicts and frustrations, as well as the hopes and fulfillments, that have gone into his life. A "good" death, therefore, is not necessarily one that is free of pain but one that retains for the individual whatever options are left to him, including the struggle to stay alive.

"I don't believe in people dying peacefully," says the clinical psychotherapist, Lawrence LeShan, who works extensively with terminal patients. "I choose to aid the patient to fight for life." Dr. LeShan calls this approach the "open encounter" and says that one's fear of death actually drops off when he struggles against dying.

Those who would expedite the dying process almost always ignore the effect of such action on survivors. Death is a social event; it involves many people. Even under favorable circumstances, the loss of a close relative usually creates feelings of "survival" guilt. In cases of sudden accidental death and suicide, it has been shown that the effects of grief and guilt are even more shattering, often leading to serious physical illness and even death among the survivors. Dr. Kutscher of the Thanatology Foundation thinks this could also be one of the dangers of the Living Will.

"The weakest link in the right to die argument," he says, "is that it neglects the alternatives. If a person can be made comfortable right up to the end, he doesn't need to be put to death." Why not, he suggests, form "life conferences" rather than death committees? Family, clergy, doctor, social worker and psychiatrist would be concerned with the patient on a daily basis, making certain that he enjoys both professional and human support in his passage from life. Emphasis would not be on ending treatment, but on strengthening the patient's morale, on making him feel wanted in this greatest and last of life's crises.

Some physicians would go further. For several years, therapists at the Maryland Psychiatric Research Center near Baltimore have used psychedelic drugs on dying patients to control the pain of some diseases and to lessen anxiety. Pioneered by the late Dr. Walter Pahnke, a Doctor of Divinity as well as an M.D., this approach seeks to give the dying patient a semimystical "peak" experience, or ecstasy—a symbolic death-and-rebirth as a preliminary to the real thing. Even when such a peak is not achieved— about two-thirds of the sixty patients who volunteered for the initial project settled for less—the therapeutic results were considered favorable.

Similar experiments at the Menninger School of Psychiatry in Topeka, Kansas, suggest that LSD does have value in alleviating the feeling of "doom and destruction" that hangs over the dying patient. The school's Dr. David V. Sheehan has reported that "patients on LSD were so strikingly unconcerned about death or any other anticipatory concern that death seemed unimportant. . . the imagery and esthetic stimulation of the drug seemed to create a new zest for experience. . ."

More conservative practitioners question the value of a "psychedelic afterglow" or an "oceanic sensation" for the dying and doubt that death can or should be made into a "trip." They argue that, just as it does with the healthy, drug-induced euphoria violates the integrity of the self and excludes the possibility of genuine experience.

With the terminally ill, what matters is not the number of days that are left but the quality of those days. Dr. LeShan, who notes that a terminal illness may last for a considerable period of time, urges his patients to do what they have always wanted to, within the limits of their situation. One man, given three months to live, decided to become a sculptor, made two trips to Italy, created several statues and lived not three months but two years—"the most important in his life," in LeShan's words.

"I tell my patients, 'Your life is worth fighting for. Sell it at the highest price you can get.'" In one instance, this advice had unexpected results. Encouraged to do his own thing, a terminal patient decided to leave his wife while he was still well enough to do so. More typical is the sixty-eight-year-old woman dying of cancer who decided to write a history of ballet. Filling her hospital room with books, playbills and newspaper clippings, she worked until the very end. "The book was not completed but her life was," LeShan says. "She died in vital contact with what she was doing."

The future of the right-to-die movement, however, may well lie with the civil libertarians rather than the medical profession. The current proliferation of "death and dying" courses in colleges, and even high schools; a fashionable insistence on dying at home; an effort to rationalize what is essentially an opaque and inexplicable experience; the effort by organized religion to reclaim the dying souls that have been lost to organized medicine; the anti-technology of present-day liberalism—all these have tipped the balance in favor of death by consent, and all in the name of a human right.

The Euthanasia Council's membership has grown five-fold in the last six years. The courts are increasingly sympathetic to the wishes of the dying patient, and the Living Will is beginning to be honored by some physicians. "Great," said one doctor in a Westchester public hospital when he first heard of it. "This makes things easier for all of us."

Skeptics are not so sure. The real right of the dying, they say—the human right—is to be treated as one of the living, with respect, good care, compassion and a measure of hope. Such an approach disturbs few consciences, minimizes risk and imposes no undue responsibility on society for deciding when people have lived long enough. The vast majority of us, even when old and ill, are in no hurry to die.

Epilogue

Life and Death:
Current Public Attitudes

John M. Ostheimer and Leonard G. Ritt

Once considered essentially medical problems, genetics, sterilization, abortion, and euthanasia are rapidly developing into political
issues. Many Americans feel that this is unfortunate; delicate
moral issues should remain private affairs, with clergy or physicians serving as advisers to personal decisions. Others believe these
questions must be considered part of the public realm. It is hard to
ignore the more sensational cases that have come to the public's
attention: poor Southern women sterilized against their will; a
doctor convicted of manslaughter for allowing a fetus to die
following an abortion; another physician indicted for murder for
not keeping a patient alive by artificial means.

None of these issues is new; they have been with us for a long
time. Compulsory sterilization has long been used as a means to
control criminality, imbecility, and other socially "unacceptable"
behavior. Geneticists and their followers felt that undesirable traits
could be avoided if successive generations of "misfits" were
removed from the pool of genetic supply. Sterilization was even
occasionally meted out as punishment. Euthanasia was (and still
is) accepted by some societies, including our own, as a way to
ensure the peaceful death of a loved one. Many Americans are
aware of the Eskimo tradition in which the aged willingly accept
their one-way trip from the igloo. Societies such as the Eskimo
have neither the extraordinary desire to maintain life far beyond
the individual's "useful" participation nor the technology to deal
with complicated medical disorders. Without malice, they have
practiced positive euthanasia. (The word means "good death.")
Abortion up to the twentieth week of pregnancy was accepted in
the United States until 1828, and then the objections were
medical (anesthesia and antiseptics were unknown) rather than
moral. Moral reasons did not become important until the second

279

half of the nineteenth century, when Anthony Comstock and others campaigned with fervor and sensationalism for very stringent abortion laws (Rockefeller Commission, 1972).

In the modern revival of these issues, the pressure of moral and ethical considerations is particularly dominant. The Prohibition experience shows that American society has difficulty in making acceptable and long-standing policies when moral issues are at stake. Thus it is particularly important to understand how the public is reacting, and what pitfalls responsible citizens must watch for if they hope to "reduce the heat" and increase the effectiveness of policy-making.

Assessing the Contemporary Significance
of Life-and-Death Issues

PUBLIC ATTITUDES

Examining public attitudes, as they have been measured by increasingly accurate mass sampling techniques, is one way to determine the importance of an issue in American society. Such a scrutiny shows that the issues discussed in this book, though undeniably gaining in importance, are still far from being general public preoccupations. As of early 1975, the "most important problems" lists published regularly in *Gallup Opinion Index, Current Opinion,* and other national poll compendiums carried no mention of these issues. But it would be wrong to use that as an excuse to dismiss them as unimportant. It took a rare person not to have been "most concerned" with Vietnam and then with the economy during the past decade. The predominance of economic issues in the public mind is especially well known. One example suffices: while 25 percent of Gallup's respondents listed inflation as the country's "most important problem" in January 1974, within eight months 81 percent of the sample were most concerned with that problem. Only a very dramatic sequence of events (along with a dearth of economic issues during a period of prosperity, perhaps) could trigger a similar reaction to the issues that are the concern of this book.

It is wiser to place "our" issues in perspective. In examining public views on questions of values, or cultural preferences ("style issues," as social scientists call them), we must bear in mind that they are usually preempted by "bread-and-butter" concerns. Table 1 indicates that awareness of abortion issues is already quite widespread; few respondents "don't know" or have "no opinion." In fact, in March of 1973 the National Opinion Research Center's annual social attitude survey found that 86 percent of the public had heard about the Supreme Court's January abortion decision. Table 1 also shows that *acceptance* of abortion had been increasing (particularly if the data on Question 4 are an indication) and that the public is becoming more inclined to accept non-medical (personal or social) justifications for abortion.

In a 1971 analysis of public opinion on abortion published in *Science,* Judith Blake stated that "a nationwide elimination of antiabortion laws would be unpopular with a majority of Americans." After so many years of pro-natalist population policies, it was only natural that public attitudes should be hostile to abortion on demand. However, Blake concluded that a liberal court ruling "would affect fewer people, and would be disapproved by no more, than any other recent social changes initiated under the impetus of judicial rulings on constitutionality" (1971:548). Four years later, (after that very Supreme court ruling in January 1973 and the growth of a vocal movement to reverse it), abortion attitude data suggest that the Court decision was more in tune with public attitudes than Blake could have known.

PROFESSIONAL ELITES

Relevant elites are already extensively involved in the abortion controversy. The Edelin abortion-manslaughter case dramatized the bitter divisions among nurses and doctors. It was probably premature to create the impression, as did Sarvis and Rodman (see Chapter 9), that medical elites are leading the movement toward acceptance of abortion; they cited evidence that psychiatrists tend increasingly to refer to abortions as "therapeutic," and that half the country's physicians favored abortion-on-request by 1970. Would doctors retain this view in the face of a revolt by their patients, if public attitudes were to turn against abortion during the middle and late 1970s? More cautiously, we may state that at the very least, attitudes within those key professional elites were showing a trend away from pronatalism.

Interest groups concerned with abortion, sterilization, and euthanasia have grown rapidly; the Euthanasia Education Council of New York has increased its membership from 600 to 30,000 in five years. Older groups—the ACLU, the U.S. Catholic Conference,

Table 1. ATTITUDES TOWARD ABORTION, 1966-74

Reason for Abortion	Response	1966	1972	1973	1974
1. Defect in the baby	yes	54%	74%	83%	83%
	no	32	20	16	14
	?	14	5	3	3
2. Mother wants no more children	yes	—	38	46	45
	no	—	58	51	51
	?	—	6	3	5
3. Mother's health threatened	yes	77	83	91	90
	no	16	13	8	8
	?	7	5	2	2
4. Family is very poor	yes	18	45	52	52
	no	72	48	45	43
	?	10	7	3	5
5. Pregnancy result of rape	yes	—	74	81	83
	no	—	20	16	13
	?	—	6	4	4
6. Mother wants to remain single	yes	—	41	47	48
	no	—	53	49	48
	?	—	7	4	4

Sources: Statistics for 1966 are from the *Gallup Opinion Index* January 1966, pp. 19-21, and represent responses to: "Do you think abortion operations should or should not be legal when. . ."
1. "the child may be born deformed?"
2. "the health of the mother is in danger?"
3. "the family does not have enough money to support another child?"

Statistics for 1972-74 are from the National Opinion Research Center (NORC), *Spring General Social Survey,* March 1972, March 1973, and March 1974 and represent responses to: "Please tell me whether or not you think it should be possible for a pregnant woman to obtain a legal abortion if. . ."
1. "there is a strong chance of serious defect in the baby?"
2. "she is married and does not want any more children?"
3. "the woman's own health is seriously endangered by the pregnancy?"
4. "the family has a very low income and cannot afford any more children?"
5. "she became pregnant as a result of rape?"
6. "she is not married and does not want to marry the man?"

the Commission on Interfaith Activities, etc.—have also given increased attention to these issues. Furthermore, the media have played a key role, giving "front page" coverage to significant cases. Books such as Stewart Alsop's *Stay of Execution,* in which the nationally known columnist spoke directly of his own impending death by cancer, have encouraged frank and open discussion of subjects once unmentionable. There is a considerable academic debate over such topics as when human life begins, and how it should end. Although not the nation's "most important problem," these issues are of growing significance in the public consciousness in large measure because of the interest they generate among professional and communications elites.

POLITICAL ELITES

The views of political elites are perhaps best studied by considering the recent activities of Congress in the realm of life and death issues. Congress has evinced a noticeable change on such issues, particularly abortion. Subsequent to the 1973 Supreme Court decision, amendments were introduced in the Senate by James Buckley (Cons., N.Y.) and Jesse Helms (R., N.C.) that would effectively have overruled the judges' decision. The Senate Judiciary Committee's Subcommittee on Constitutional Amendments held hearings throughout 1974, but took no action. In the House, Congressmen Don Edwards' (D., Calif.) view prevailed: there was not sufficient interest for his Judiciary subcommittee to hold hearings.

In both houses, a number of other political questions were involved in all the recent abortion votes: thus it is not that simple to isolate Congress' attitudes on abortion specifically. In 1973, both the House and the Senate passed amendments to measures providing legal services for the poor which would have barred the Legal Services Corporation from funding abortions. Lawrence Hogan's (R., Md.) amendment, introduced on June 21, 1973, was further amended by Harold Froelich (R., Wisc.), to prohibit poverty lawyers from helping a woman obtain a therapeutic abortion if doing so was against the woman's convictions. This package passed overwhelmingly and was subsequently adopted by voice vote in the Senate. In May 1974, that broad legislation which included the ban against involuntary abortions was accepted by both houses. It was signed into law July 25, 1974.

The abortion issue also arose when Congress considered

extending the OEO Program in May 1974. The House accepted two amendments: one proposed by Froelich to bar the use of community action funds for medical assistance and supplies in abortion cases, the other to ban the use of those same funds for sterilizations.

Then, reversing its previous stands, on June 27, 1974 the House rejected (123-247) an amendment introduced by Angelo Roncallo (R., N.Y.) that would have prohibited the use of HEW Funds for abortions or abortion-related matters. Roncallo contended that HEW was already funding abortions. He cited evidence that in New York State, 27,000 abortions at a cost of $2.7 million in medicaid payments had been carried out over a 15-month period. Some observers argued that the lateness of the hour when the issue reached a vote may have contributed to its defeat (*Congressional Quarterly:* July 6, 1974, 1969). Their assertion might be questioned in light of a subsequent event. When the House of Representatives discussed committee reform on October 8, 1974, Froelich proposed that a special legislative committee be set up to investigate the problem of abortion. His motion was defeated 163-193. These last two votes suggest that the House had begun to respond to the growing permissiveness toward abortion-on-demand revealed in the public opinion surveys. Thus, at the elite level, the issue may be losing its volatility as long as there is no question of governmental coercion.

In the Senate, Dewey Bartlett (R., Okla.) led a battle similar to Roncallo's on the HEW Appropriations Bill. On September 17, 1974, the Senate accepted his anti-abortion amendment by voice vote after refusing 34-50 to table it. Bartlett estimated that HEW had spent $40-50 million nationally in 1973 under medicaid to pay for about 270,000 abortions. His amendment was dropped from the final bill by Senate-House conferees, but Bartlett resurrected it on April 10, 1975 in connection with a health and nurse training bill. This time his amendment was tabled (and thus defeated) by a vote of 54-36. The opposition was led by Senator Edward Kennedy (D., Mass.) who up to that time had maintained a low profile on the issue. Stating that he opposed abortion, Kennedy argued that his personal views were, however, irrelevant: the amendment was illegal because courts had held that if the federal government pays for prenatal and maternity care, it must also pay for abortions.

Although most attention in the 93rd Congress was focused on

abortion, Senator Kennedy held hearings in 1973 concerning experiments on fetuses and human beings. Furthermore, there were revelations of research employing psychosurgery, as well as other experiments using children, prisoners, and the mentally retarded. These matters came up in the Senate, but the first votes on the issue came in the House when it considered the NSF funding bill. On April 18, 1974, the House rejected a lenient version of an amendment which would have allowed fetal experimentation if it was carried out in furtherance of "the duties and responsibilities of the medical profession." As this wording suggests, the researcher's own judgment was to be the foremost factor in his decision. The House then forbade *any* experimentation on human fetuses by a vote of 281-58. Both amendments were offered by Representative Roncallo. Anti-abortion groups had indicated that these votes were measures of the political strength of their opponents. The Senate on May 16, 1974 passed an NSF funding bill without the House ban. But the final bill which cleared Congress (June 28, 1974) created a temporary commission to oversee the use of human subjects in medical experimentation, and it banned HEW-funded research in the area.

For reasons not altogether clear, the House made a substantial turnabout on the abortion issue during May-June 1974. Before May 1974, opposition to restricting the federal government's role in funding abortions came mainly from a small group of Northern Democrats. Support for such restrictions came from the familiar "conservative coalition" of Republicans and Southern Democrats. Approximately the same set of alliances appeared on the fetal research amendment. After June 1974, however, the conservative coalition began to disintegrate. Seventy percent of the Republicans supported the Froelich Amendment to set up a special committee to study abortion; but a majority of Southern Democrats joined with a majority of Northern Democrats to defeat the proposal. In fact, 85 percent of the Southern Democrats, as opposed to 58 percent of the Northern Democrats, voted against the amendment. The votes of Northern Catholic representatives are particularly interesting. Preliminary analyses suggest that whereas Catholic Democrats in Congress split about even, 82 percent of the Catholic Republican representatives were anti-abortion. Similar partisan patterns exist within other denominational groups, suggesting that among legislators party is becoming more important than religious background.

In the Senate a rather dramatic reversal took place between June 1974 and April 1975 on the Bartlett anti-abortion amendment. On the first vote, the more lenient position was supported by Northern Democrats (50 percent) plus a substantial minority of Republicans (39 percent). Southern Democrats, on the other hand, supported the hard-line amendment overwhelmingly (83 percent), as did most Catholic Senators, with the notable exception of Senator Kennedy. By April 1975, most of the vote switching had come from Catholic Northern Democrats (Muskie, Mansfield, McIntyre) and Southerners (Nunn, Huddleston, Byrd). Thus, in the Senate as in the House, it would seem that support for more lenient abortion attitudes is becoming a Democratic partisan stance.

Variations in Public Reaction

Unlike legislators, most Americans have not had to express publicly their own views on abortion or related issues. And not all Americans have been similarly affected by, or are equally conscious of, life and death concerns. (Table 2 indicates only the percentage of the sample "in agreement" with abortion and/or euthanasia. "No opinion" responses to the euthanasia question, not shown in that table, ran 7 percent for the nation as a whole, but were as high as 17 percent among farmers.) Urban, more educated, white-collar, and younger respondents were more apt to have an opinion. These patterns were repeated on the abortion question used to compile Table 2, with "no opinion" highest among nonwhites, people over fifty, and Westerners.

As for euthanasia, represented in Table 2 by a question that implies positive action by the physician, the results indicate that education and age are very strongly related to acceptance of the concept. One should note also that people over fifty were by 1973 almost evenly divided (44 percent "yes," 47 percent "no," 9 percent "no opinion") on an issue that becomes increasingly salient with age.

Other poll data cast some doubt on the assumption that euthanasia is achieving widespread public acceptance. Table 3 shows the results of a March 1973 Harris Poll that included one question suggesting positive euthanasia, another a more passive concept of simply ceasing to use medical treatment to extend life. It seems that the distinction between the two forms of euthanasia *is* perceived by the public, and is still very much a factor in

Table 2. ATTITUDES TOWARD EUTHANASIA AND ABORTION, 1950-74
(Respondents favoring the more permissive attitude)

| | Euthanasia | | Abortion | |
	1950	1973	1969	1974
National sample	36%	53%	40%	47%
Sex				
Men	38	53	50	51
Women	34	53	40	43
Education				
College	42	61	58	67
High school	39	54	37	44
Grade school	31	39	31	25
Age				
Under 30	39	67	46	55
30-49	37	51	39	44
50 and over	30	44	38	43
Race				
White	—	54	40	47
Nonwhite	—	53	45	45
Occupation				
Professional and business	—	58	52	59
White collar	—	63	40	54
Farmers	—	42	38	—
Manual workers	—	52	35	44
Nonlabor force	—	—	—	40
Religion				
Protestant	36[a]	52[a]	40	48
Catholic	28[a]	46[a]	31	32
Jew	54[a]	60[a]	—	—
Politics				
Republicans	—	50	46	49
Democrats	—	49	35	42
Independents	—	49	42	52

continued on next page

Table 2 (continued)

Region	Euthanasia		Abortion	
	1950	1973	1969	1974
East	—	51	45	52
Midwest	—	51	37	41
South	—	48	33	39
West	—	64	48	59
Income				
$20,000 and over	—	—	—	60
$15,000 and over	—	60	54	49
$10,000-14,999	—	54	44	44
$7,000-9,999	—	48	43	41
$5,000-6,999	—	55	34	42
$3,000-4,999	—	46	31	49
under $3,000	—	45	33	27
Community size				
1 million and over	—	52	53	58
500,000-999,999	—	55	53	51
50,000-499,999	—	n.a.	39	50
2,500-49,000	—	53	31	44
Under 2,500 (rural)	—	48	32	36
Marital Status				
Married	—	—	—	46
Single	—	—	—	56

Sources: Statistics on euthanasia, 1950 and 1973, are from the *Gallup Opinion Index,* August 1973, pp. 35-37, and represent positive responses to the question: "When a person has a disease that cannot be cured, do you think doctors should be allowed by law to end the patient's life by some painless means if the patient and his family request it?"

Statistics on abortion for 1969 are from the *Gallup Opinion Index,* December 1969, p. 19, and represent favorable responses to the question: "Would you favor or oppose a law which would permit a woman to go to a doctor to end a pregnancy at any time during the first three months?"

Statistics on abortion for 1974 are from the *Gallup Opinion Index,* April 1974, p. 24, and represent favorable responses to the question: "The U.S. Supreme Court has ruled that a woman may go to a doctor to end pregnancy at any time during the first three months of pregnancy. Do you favor or oppose this ruling?"

[a]Data reported by *Current Opinion* (April 1974), p. 39, as taken from Gallup polls of 1947 and 1973.

determining public reaction. Of course, without standardization of the polling question, it is difficult to determine precisely what the public thinks: Gallup's July 1973 "end the patient's life" (Table 2, 53 percent approve) drew a response very different from Harris's March 1973 "put him out of his misery" (Table 3, 37 percent approve).

No poll data exist regarding compulsory sterilization or eugenic manipulation, but attitude data on abortion show some similar trends (as noted in our discussion of Table 1), as well as some trends that differ from those indicated in the euthanasia responses. Religion is perhaps the most interesting category, because so very much has been said about the role of Roman Catholicism in the organizations and lobbying efforts that have followed the Supreme Court's decision. Judith Blake's article in *Science,* the most exhaustive recent writing on abortion-related attitudes, was dominated by the theme of Catholic-Protestant division, though she concluded that the attitudes of Catholics and Protestants are closer than one might expect "when one considers that the Catholic Church unconditionally bans the induced termination of pregnancy." She added, and the more recent data presented below confirm, that "It is an exaggeration to think of American Catholics as representing, in fact, a blueprint of church doctrine." (1971:547).

Table 3. CONTRASTING ATTITUDES TOWARD "POSITIVE" AND
          "PASSIVE" EUTHANASIA

Attitude	1. Passive Euthanasia	2. Positive Euthanasia
"Ought to be allowed"	62%	37%
"It is wrong"	28	53
"Not sure"	10	10

Source: Current Opinion (June 1973), p. 60. Statistics are from a Harris Poll, March 1973, and represent responses to the questions:

1. "Do you think a patient with a terminal disease ought to be able to tell his doctor to let him die rather than to extend his life when cure is in sight, or do you think this is wrong?"

2. "Do you think the patient who is terminally ill, with no cure in sight, ought to have the right to tell his doctor to put him out of his misery, or do you think this is wrong?"

Table 4. RESPONDENTS FAVORING ABORTION FOR MEDICAL AND PERSONAL REASONS,
BY CATEGORIES OF AND STRENGTH OF RELIGION

Reasons for Favoring Abortion	Catholics	Jews	Protestants	Baptists	Methodists	Lutherans	Presybterians	Episcopalians
Medical Reasons								
Strong religion	54%	100%	66%	60%	80%	71%	93%	95%
Not very strong	82	100	80	70	80	87	89	79
Personal Reasons								
Strong religion	18	86	27	19	40	21	59	58
Not very strong	42	79	41	29	42	55	50	58

Sources: See Table 1. "Medical reasons" are composite scores, respondents in agreement with question 1, 3, and 5.
"Personal reasons" are composite scores for questions 2, 4, and 6.
Strength of religion is measured by the question, "Would you consider yourself a strong or a not very strong (religious or denominational preference)?"

It is unfortunate that Blake's data did not permit analysis of the *intensity* of religious feelings, or of the differences between various Protestant denominations. The overall role of religion in shaping attitudes toward abortion (and presumably toward other life and death issues) seems no less significant than it was several years ago, but our data show that the divisions are not so simple as "Protestant vs. Catholic." Table 4 is based on two composite scales, rather than the six separate questions given in Table 1. In this method, which simplified analysis, the three questions justifying abortion on medical grounds (Questions 1, 3, and 5, in Table 1) were combined, as were the three "non-medical" or personal reasons. Obviously, strength of religious belief is dramatically associated with opposition to abortion. Most notably, the Catholic sub-sample shows a far stronger tendency to move toward acceptance as intensity of religious feelings declines: where "strong" Catholics are less tolerant of abortion than are "strong" Protestants, weaker Catholics are at least as accepting as weaker Protestants, and weak Catholics are more permissive than are strong Protestants.

The same picture emerges for various Protestant denominations. Members of the more fundamentalist denominations, however, do not seem to vary in their opinions according to the intensity of their religion: "weak" Baptists are less in favor of abortion than are "weak" Catholics, and nearly as opposed as "strong" Catholics.

Since holding strength of religion constant fails to reduce the differences between religions, one might argue that education is logically the key determinant in abortion attitudes. Catholics and Baptists tend to be lower socioeconomic-status groups, and their class status affects their stance on abortion. To determine whether religion or education is the more powerful descriptor, educational levels of respondents were held constant. Table 5 shows that strong differences divide Protestant denominations even at higher education categories; Baptists are just as opposed to abortion as Catholics. (Throughout the analysis, the Jewish sub-sample was too small to allow rigorous analysis, but Jews were the group most strongly favoring abortion. Their support was ordinarily stronger even than respondents who had "no religion".) Although educational level has comparatively little impact on the attitudes of Baptists or Catholics toward abortion for personal reasons, more educated Baptists are more likely to favor abortion for medical reasons.

Table 5. RESPONDENTS FAVORING ABORTION FOR MEDICAL AND PERSONAL REASONS, BY RELIGION AND EDUCATION

Reasons for Favoring Abortion	No religion	Jews	Catholics	Protestants	Baptists	Methodists	Lutherans	Presbyterians	Episcopalians
Medical reasons									
Grade school only	73%	100%	65%	62%	57%	68%	37%	77%	71%
High school graduates	87	100	72	79	71	84	83	91	83
College graduates	100	100	68	90	89	92	93	92	100
Personal reasons									
Grade school only	33	44	29	25	20	32	30	31	29
High school graduates	66	94	31	37	26	41	44	46	61
College graduates	83	89	38	58	39	65	57	73	69

Sources: See Table 4.

Another noteworthy trend identifiable in Table 5 is that, though the overall difference between Protestant denominations is confirmed, education emerges as an important indicator in its own right. Low education is associated with low tolerance for abortion among all denominations. The prospects of liberalized public response to abortion (and presumably for other life and death issues as well) should be seen as a function of the publicity given to the issue. When elites have become fully informed, and when other issues have subsided, abortion and other life and death issues will receive more attention from a communications system dominated by more liberal elites; their favorable attitudes will exert a liberal pull on the middle and lower educational levels. Blake's analysis of earlier poll data demonstrated that even during the 1960s, when "pro-natalist" attitudes were stronger than at present, the most substantial change toward accepting personal, non-medical grounds for abortion was the 20 percent shift by white, non-Catholic, college-educated men. That shift was especially significant because the group in question constitutes a disproportionately powerful sector of the population.

One proviso concerning the apparent impact of education is in order. We had reason to expect that race differences might explain some variations among attitudes toward abortion. Sections of the black elite in the United States (Gregory, 1971; Ostheimer and Ritt, 1975) and for that matter throughout the black world (*Africa Report*, 1974) have labelled such activities as sterilization, family planning clinics and the entire population control movement advocated by environmentalists as "genocide." We have found some confirmation for the hypothesis that the black perspective, at least among the black elite, appears to affect attitudes toward abortion. Table 6 shows that among blacks higher education is *not* as strongly associated with a continued increase in acceptance of abortion as it is among whites. Nor, interestingly, are there differences among blacks of varying religions or denominations.

The political "location" of life and death issues in federalized America, with its regional differences and local bases of political power, is surprisingly hard to determine. It is not easy to label "pro-life" forces as Democratic or Republican; nor can the partisan identity of abortion or euthanasia advocates, or other camps on the opposite side of the issues, be easily pinned down. Table 7 shows Republicans generally in favor of abortion and

Table 6. RESPONDENTS FAVORING ABORTION FOR MEDICAL
AND PERSONAL REASONS, BY RACE, CONTROLLING
SEPARATELY FOR EDUCATION AND RELIGION

Reasons for Favoring Abortion	*Blacks*	*Whites*
Medical reasons		
Grade school only	39%	69%
High school graduates	74	78
College graduates	69	88
Catholics	92	77
Protestants (combined)	78	88
Baptists	81	84
Methodists	84	90
Personal reasons		
Grade school only	20	28
High school graduates	25	39
College graduates	39	54
Catholics	46	39
Protestants (combined)	36	47
Baptists	37	33
Methodists	42	52

Source: See Table 4.

euthanasia. But key groups who advocate that stance—for example, women's rights organizations—are usually more identified with the Democratic party. To complicate the picture further, Catholics, ordinarily more likely to be Democrats, generally oppose abortion, and another strong Democratic Party bloc, the black masses, do not notably diverge from the national attitude trends, despite the campaign by at least some black intellectuals to label such policies "genocide." On the other hand, the Democratic Party's liberal-intellectual elements are distinctly favorably inclined. (Note, for example, Jewish attitudes.) Thus at this stage, one can make few strong statements connecting opinions on life and death issues to political party. Liberal Democrats are balanced by Southern and blue-collar elements. On the Republican side, conservative, traditionalist, and farmer elements are balanced by high socioeconomic status Republican moderates.

The National Opinion Research Center's data suggest that self-perceived ideology is a more powerful indicator of abortion attitudes than is political party. Table 7 suggests that permissive abortion laws emerge as a "liberal" cause particularly among higher educated liberals, especially in the case of abortion for social or personal reasons.

Table 7 further shows that religion holds its power to separate Americans into distinct groups, as far as their attitudes on abortion are concerned, even when key political variables are held constant. Baptists and Catholics are uniformly less willing to accept abortion than are others, regardless of their political party affiliation, ideological self-identification, or vote in 1972. It seems particularly interesting that "conservatives" from most denominations are more often in favor of abortion than are "liberal" Baptists.

There are two obvious explanations for the power of religion. First, religion is understandably an important determinant in any moral issue. But to understand why political variables do not account for large variations in abortion attitudes, one must recognize that even abortion, the most well publicized of life and death matters, has not had time to become established in the popular mind as a partisan issue. This relative newness of abortion as a political controversy may also explain the tendency of political variables to break down in comparison with educational levels. Table 8 shows that less educated Republicans and Democrats share closer attitudes on abortion than do Republicans (or Democrats) at different educational levels.

Ideological labels also fail to predict abortion attitudes. Being "conservative" or "liberal" seems to count for less than does educational level, though when personal reasons are the justification for abortion, well-educated conservatives are much slower to accept the more permissive stance.

Of the political variables, Presidential vote in 1972 seems to have the strongest relationship with abortion attitudes, but its direction is curious, to say the least. One of the more vivid differences between Nixon and McGovern was on cultural issues such as marijuana, amnesty and abortion. Yet, according to the National Opinion Research Center's sample, Nixon voters were more permissive; in four of the six categories of education-abortion attitude, Nixon voters were notably more pro-abortion. A possible interpretation of this finding is that McGovern drew

Table 7. RESPONDENTS FAVORING ABORTION FOR MEDICAL AND PERSONAL REASONS, BY RELIGION AND POLITICAL VARIABLES

Reasons for Favoring Abortion	No religion	Catholics	Protestants	Baptists	Methodists	Lutherans	Presbyterians	Episcopalians
Medical reasons								
Democrats	90%	65%	72%	67%	83%	80%	70%	78%
Independents	83	76	77	72	74	97	89	89
Republicans	88	68	76	59	82	71	96	97
McGovern voters	88	69	71	67	71	75	100	100
Nixon voters	95	67	82	72	82	88	93	96
Liberals	86	71	76	64	89	78	100	100
Moderates	90	74	78	73	81	89	85	81
Conservatives	73	58	74	67	75	77	87	82
Personal reasons								
Democrats	73	27	30	21	38	35	53	56
Independents	58	38	41	33	39	53	57	44
Republicans	63	32	37	23	45	38	44	71
McGovern voters	66	35	36	22	39	40	65	100
Nixon voters	81	28	41	32	46	46	52	70
Liberals	71	39	42	29	55	57	71	70
Moderates	48	32	34	28	40	34	42	44
Conservatives	57	22	36	20	39	40	52	64

Source: See Table 4.

Table 8. RESPONDENTS FAVORING ABORTION FOR MEDICAL AND
PERSONAL REASONS, BY POLITICAL VARIABLES,
CONTROLLING FOR EDUCATION

Reasons for Favoring Abortion	Grade School Only	High School Graduates	College Graduates
Medical reasons			
Democrats	64%	76%	89%
Independents	72	80	82
Republicans	57	80	92
McGovern voters	59	78	87
Nixon voters	72	80	89
Liberals	60	84	91
Moderates	68	84	85
Conservatives	67	67	84
Personal reasons			
Democrats	26	33	68
Independents	34	42	55
Republicans	20	42	25
McGovern voters	26	38	40
Nixon voters	32	62	60
Liberals	30	49	72
Moderates	28	36	59
Conservatives	26	33	43

Source: See Table 4.

strong support from the traditional Democratic constituency,
many of whom are Catholic and black; these voters ignored
McGovern's cultural issue stands because of their agreement with
his economic positions, which were more directly related to their
daily lives.

Religion has a greater effect on 1972 vote than does education.
For example, in Table 7, McGovernite Baptists had more in
common with Nixonite Baptists on abortion issues than they did
with McGovernite Presbyterians. Education's impact seems to have
been similar to that of religion, but simply not as strong. Indeed, it
loses its impact at the two higher education categories where the
Nixon voters were, curiously, so relatively pro-abortion.

Conclusions

Our analysis has returned to the first topic of the chapter, the prominence of life and death issues in the general public consciousness. It is obvious that the role of religion is closely associated with public attitudes, but education can weaken "pro-natalism." Educated elites are the first to react favorably to abortion and euthanasia, and, presumably, to sterilization and eugenic change. But as broader masses of the public become more concerned about the issues, their reaction may not be as positive. Strong Catholic and Baptist beliefs are likely to promote hostility to the liberal movements, and generate support for "right-to-life" causes.

Politically, life and death issues may cause yet another internal conflict in the Democratic Party, that fragile patchwork that provides both the intellectual leadership for "modernistic attitudes" on such issues, and the mass Catholic and Baptist support for the attack against them. The political nature of the issues is not yet clearly identified, but when the key issues of the late 1960s and early 1970s subside, life and death concerns will surely move into the political spotlight.

References

Africa Report (July, August 1974).

Blake, Judith, "Abortion and Public Opinion: the 1960-1970 Decade," *Science* 171 (February 12, 1971) 540-549.

Gregory, D. "My Answer to Genocide," *Ebony* (October 1971), 66-72.

National Opinion Research Center, *Spring 1974 General Social Survey* (Williamstown, Mass: Roper Public Opinion Research Center, 1974).

Ostheimer, John M. and Leonard G. Ritt, "Environment, Energy and Black Americans," (Beverly Hills, CA: Sage Research Papers in the Social Sciences—Human Ecology Series, #90-025, 1975).

Rockefeller Commission on Population Growth and the American Future, *Population and the American Future* (New York: Signet, 1972).

Sarvis, Betty, and Hyman Rodman, *The Abortion Controversy* (New York: Columbia University Press, 1973).

The authors wish to thank Transition Foundation of Los Angeles for financial assistance supporting the research for the epilogue.

Further Readings

General

Albertson, Peter, and M. Barnett. *Managing the Planet*. Englewood Cliffs, N.J.: Prentice-Hall, 1972.

Alsop, Stewart. *Stay of Execution*. Philadelphia: Lippincott, 1973.

Ardrey, Robert. *The Social Contract*. New York: Atheneum, 1970.

The Commission on Population Growth and the American Future. *Population and the American Future*. New York: New American Library, 1972.

Ehrlich, Paul R. *The Population Bomb*. New York: Ballantine, 1971.

Francoer, R.T. "Utopian Motherhood and Population Control." *Catalyst for Environmental Quality* 1 (1971), pp. 7-10.

Jacker, Corinne. *The Biological Revolution*. New York: Parents Magazine Press, 1971.

Ramparts editors. *Eco-catastrophe*. San Francisco: Canfield Press, 1970.

Sherman, Adams E. "Unwanted Births and Poverty in the United States." *The Conference Board Record* 6:4 (1969), pp. 10-17.

Skinner, B.F. *Beyond Freedom and Dignity*. New York: Bantam, 1972.

Teilhard de Chardin, Pierre. *The Phenomenon of Man*. New York: Harper, 1959.

Eugenics: Social Choice or Nature's Way?

Ausebel, F., J. Beckwith, and K. Janssen. "The Politics of Genetic Engineering: Who Decides Who's Defective?" *Psychology Today*, June 1974, pp. 30-43.

Bresler, Jack B., ed. *Genetics and Society*. Reading, Mass.: Addison-Wesley, 1973.

Callahan, Daniel. *The Tyranny of Survival*. New York: Macmillan, 1973.

Carlson, E.A., "H.J. Muller." *Genetics* 70 (1972), pp. 1-30.

Dunn, Leslie C., and T. Dobzhansky. *Heredity, Race and Society*. New York: New American Library, 1952.

English, D.S., "Genetic Manipulation and Man." *The American Biology Teacher* 34 (1972), pp. 507-14.

_____. *Genetic and Reproductive Engineering.* New York: MSS Information Corporation, 1974.

Etzioni, Amitai. *Genetic Fix.* New York: Macmillan, 1973.

Fasten, N., *Principles of Genetics and Eugenics.* New York: Ginn, 1935.

Galton, F. *Essays on Eugenics.* London: Eugenics Education Society, 1909.

Gaylin, W. "We Have the Awful Knowledge to Make Exact Copies of Human Beings: The Frankenstein Myth Becomes a Reality." *The New York Times Magazine,* March 5, 1972, pp. 88-97.

Ludmerer, Kenneth M., *Genetics and American Society.* Baltimore: Johns Hopkins, 1972.

Merril, C.R., M.R. Geier, and J.C. Petricciani. "Bacterial Versus Gene Expression in Human Cells," *Nature* 233 (1971), pp. 398-400.

Pai, A.C. *Foundations of Genetics: A Science for Society.* New York: McGraw-Hill, 1974.

Paoletti, Robert A., ed. *Selected Readings: Genetic Engineering and Bioethics.* New York: MSS Information Corporation, 1972.

Robitsher, Jonas, ed. *Eugenic Sterilization.* Springfield, Ill.: Thomas, 1973.

Swanson, H.D. *Human Reproduction: Biology and Social Change.* London: Oxford University Press, 1974.

Taylor, Gordon R. *The Biological Time Bomb.* New York: New American Library, 1968.

Abortion on Demand

"The Abortion Dilemma." *Atlas World Press Review* 21:10 (November 1974), pp. 11-20.

Bluford, Robert, and R.E. Petres. *Unwanted Pregnancy.* New York: Harper, 1973.

Callahan, Daniel. *Abortion: Law, Choice and Morality.* New York: Macmillan, 1971.

Carmen, Arlene, and Howard Moody. *Abortion Counseling and Social Change.* Valley Forge, Pa.: Judson Press, 1973.

Carroll, Rev. Charles. "Medicine Without an Ethic." *Journal of the Louisiana State Medical Society* 124 (September 1972), pp. 313-20.

Granfield, David. *The Abortion Decision.* New York: Doubleday, 1969.

Hardin, Garrett. *Stalking the Wild Taboo.* Los Altos, Calif.: W. Kaufman, 1973.

Hilger, Thomas W., and D.J. Horan, eds. *Abortion and Social Justice.* New York: Sheed & Ward, 1972.

Hudson, R.A., H.H. Werley, J.W. Ager and F.P. Shea. "Health Professionals' Attitudes Toward Abortion." *Public Opinion Quarterly,* 1974.

Knowles, John H. "Public Policy on Abortion." *Society* 11 (July/August 1974), pp. 15-18.

Lader, Lawrence. *Abortion II: Making the Revolution.* Boston: Beacon, 1973.

Noonan, John T., Jr. *The Morality of Abortion: Legal and Historical Perspectives.* Cambridge: Harvard University Press, 1970.

Planned Parenthood of New York City. *Abortion: A Woman's Guide.* New York: Abelard-Schuman, 1973.

Reiterman, Carl, ed. *Abortion and the Unwanted Child.* New York: Springer, 1971.

van der Tak, Jean, *Abortion, Fertility, and Changing Legislation: An International Review.* (Transnational Family Research Institute), Lexington, Md.: Lexington Books, 1974.

Walbert, David F. and J.D. Butler, eds. *Abortion, Society, and the Law.* Cleveland, Ohio: Case Western Reserve Press, 1973.

Whitehead, K.D. *Catholics United for the Faith.* New Rochelle, New York: 1972.

Willke, Jack C., and Mrs. J.C. Willke. *Handbook on Abortion.* Cincinnati: Hiltz, 1971.

Compulsory Sterilization

Babcock, Richard F., Jr. "Sterilization: Coercing Consent." *The Nation,* January 12, 1974, pp. 51-53.

Barnett, Larry D. "Population Policy: Payments for Fertility Limitation in the United States." *Social Biology* 16 (December 1969).

———. "Zero Population Growth, Inc." *Bioscience* 21 (July 15, 1971), pp. 759-66.

Becker, Harold, G.T. Felkenes, and P.W. Whisenard. *New Dimensions in Criminal Justice.* Metuchen, N.J.: Scarecrow Press, 1968.

Behrman, S.J., L. Corsa, Jr., and R. Freedman, eds. *Fertility and Family Planning: A World View.* Ann Arbor: University of Michigan Press, 1969.

Berelson, Bernard. "Beyond Family Planning." *Science* 163 (1969), pp. 533-43.

Berelson, Bernard, et al. *Family Planning and Population Programs.* Chicago: University of Chicago Press, 1966.

Callahan, Daniel, ed. *The American Population Debate.* New York: Anchor/Doubleday, 1971.

Gosney, E.S., and P. Popenoe. *Sterilization for Human Betterment.* New York: Macmillan, 1929.

Lader, Lawrence, ed. *Foolproof Birth Control: Male and Female Sterilization.* Boston: Beacon, 1972.

The New York Times, "Sterilization of Black Mother of Two Stirs Aiken, S.C." August 1, 1973.

How To Die: Euthanasia

Downing, A.B., ed. *Euthanasia and the Right to Death.* London: Peter Owen, 1969.

Fletcher, Joseph. *Morals and Medicine.* Princeton: Princeton University Press, 1954.

Haering, Bernard. *Medical Ethics.* Notre Dame, Indiana: Fides, 1973.

Keleman, Stanley. *Living Your Dying.* New York: Random House/Bookworks, 1975.

Kohl, Marvin. *The Morality of Killing.* New York: Humanities Press, 1974.

Kübler-Ross, Elisabeth. *On Death and Dying.* New York: Macmillan, 1969.

Maguire, Daniel C. "Death by Chance, Death by Choice." *The Atlantic,* January 1974, pp. 57-65.

_____. "Death, Legal and Illegal." *The Atlantic,* February 1974, pp. 72-85.

"Ohioans Divided on Mercy Killing." *Current Opinion,* July 1974, p. 75.

Trubo, Richard. *An Act of Mercy: Euthanasia Today.* Los Angeles: Nash, 1973.

U.S. Senate. *Death With Dignity: An Inquiry into Related Public Issues.* (Hearings before the Special Committee on Aging, 92nd Congress, 2nd session.) Washington: U.S. Government Printing Office, 1972.

Williams, Glanville. *The Sanctity of Life and the Criminal Law.* London: Faber, 1957.

Williams, Robert, ed. *To Live and to Die: When, Why and How.* New York: Springer-Verlag, 1973.

Index

119-44